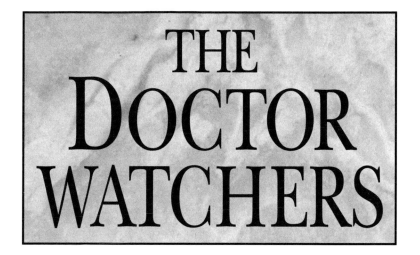

THE
DOCTOR
WATCHERS

SPENCER VIBBERT

THE GRAND ROUNDS PRESS

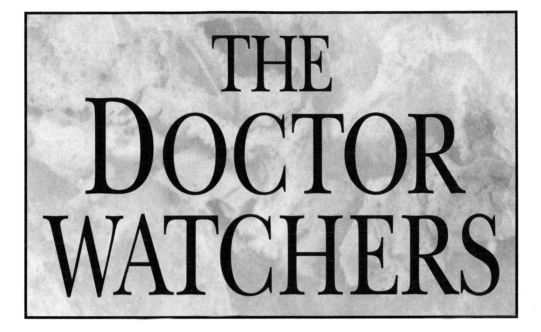

THE DOCTOR WATCHERS

SPENCER VIBBERT

WHITTLE DIRECT BOOKS

Photographs: Representative Ted Weiss: Terry Ashe/Gamma Liaison, page 2; Thomas Dehn, M.D., by David Schlabowske, page 4; William Moncrief, M.D., by Jeffery Newbury, page 5; William Diefenbach, M.D.: courtesy of Martha Diefenbach, page 8; James Patton by Breton Littlehales, page 10; Richard Kusserow: Cynthia Johnson/*Time* magazine, page 12; Senator John Heinz: courtesy of Senator Heinz's office, page 18; Thomas Morford by Max Hirschfeld, page 22; Gail Wilensky: Breton Littlehales, page 25; Andrew Webber: Charles Borniger, page 26; James Todd, M.D.: Kevin Horan, page 27; James Sammons, M.D., by Paul Elledge, page 28; John Kelly, M.D.: courtesy of John Kelly, page 32; Alice Gosfield by Sal DiMarco Jr./Black Star, page 41; Laurie Dozier, M.D., by Mark Gooch, page 55; Monsignor Charles Fahey: courtesy of Fordham University, page 60; Dennis O'Leary, M.D.: courtesy of Dennis O'Leary, page 62; Grant Rodkey, M.D.: Stella Johnson, page 63. Charts: James Stoecker, pages 17, 33, 47, 49.

Library of Congress Card Number: 91-065027
Vibbert, Spencer
The Doctor Watchers
ISBN 0-9624745-8-4
ISSN 1053-6620

The Grand Rounds Press

The Grand Rounds Press presents original short books by distinguished authors on subjects of importance to the medical profession.

The series is edited and published by Whittle Direct Books, a business unit of Whittle Communications L.P. A new book will be published approximately every three months. The series will reflect a broad spectrum of responsible opinions. In each book the opinions expressed are those of the author, not the publisher or the advertiser

We welcome your comments on this unique endeavor

CONTENTS

CHAPTER ONE

REVIEWING
THE REVIEWERS

P eer review organizations (PROs) have been scrutinizing hospital treatment of Medicare patients for more than seven years. Millions of records have been reviewed in an effort to ensure that the care the elderly are receiving is appropriate and of high quality. Yet wide disagreement remains about what, if anything, the federally funded PRO program has accomplished. The groups that lobby in Washington on PRO issues are unable to agree on what to measure—on how review entities should themselves be reviewed. Debate is muddied by emotion, politics, and self-interest. But even if no one can agree on which yardstick to use, almost everyone is united in declaring that the program has come up short.

Organized medicine has never accepted the program's premise and perhaps never will, even though PROs' rulings are ultimately made by physicians. Doctors who gather for the American Medical Association's twice-yearly House of Delegates meetings say PROs have failed in what should be their main purpose: education. Instead of teaching physicians to practice better medicine, delegates say, PROs have come to exemplify the "hassle factor"—forced compliance with an ever-expanding array of forms, procedures, and regulations. Worse yet, PROs are accused of micromanaging treatment decisions that should be left to physicians.

Epidemiologists and analysts looking for statistical evidence of change in physicians' behavior fault PROs for very different reasons. The number-crunchers complain that the program's emphasis on reviewing individual medical records leaves few resources to study broad patterns of care or to conduct population-based analyses. The success or failure of a quality-review system, these critics say, ought to be measured by its effect on patient care and on institutions' internal quality-assurance efforts, not on its ability to ferret out a few aberrant practitioners.

These same critics question the credentials of program managers at the Health Care Financing Administration (HCFA) and point to evidence of unscientific and apparently scattershot methods at the agency. What, they ask, are the qualifications of the government "experts" responsible for the anemic Preprocedure Review Program? After looking at more than 1.7 million procedure requests, this congressionally mandated cost-cutting program has produced an almost undetectable denial rate of 0.17 percent. The critics charge that no program designed by competent professionals and following sound review criteria could have produced such a dismal result.

Lists of PRO deficiencies also come from Richard Kusserow, the inspector general (IG) of the federal Department of Health and Human Services (HHS), and from lawmakers such as Representative Ted Weiss (D-N.Y.). PROs have fallen short, say these observers, because they lack the courage to attack substandard and inefficient care. As evidence, these and other government critics cite statistics from rereviews of PRO records by HCFA's so-called superPRO, SysteMetrics, a subsidiary of McGraw-Hill, which has a contract to rereview PRO findings for accuracy. SysteMetrics consistently finds defects in four to five times more cases than the PROs do. Spokespersons for the latter are quick to point out that the super-PRO isn't required to contact the treating physician before issuing a denial. This argument has swayed neither Weiss nor the IG; they retort that even when PROs find unquestionably poor care, the agencies are often extremely slow to act.

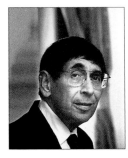

Congressman Ted Weiss, a PRO critic.

Overall, there is little statistical evidence that peer review has had much impact on Medicare spending. In addition to poor results with preprocedure review, PROs denied just 0.70 percent of ambulatory-surgery payments between April 1989, when the third scope of work became effective, and the end of the year. And while their 2.01 percent denial rate for inpatient hospital reviews might suggest that the PRO system has had some impact on hospital costs, that rate doesn't reflect subsequent reversals and modifications. Because about a quarter of denials are challenged, and 44 percent of those challenged are reversed or modified, the final inpatient hospital payment denial rate is something less than 2 percent.

Nor is the program having a clear impact on quality. Though PROs found "confirmed quality problems" in 2.32 percent of records reviewed under the third scope in 1989, the vast majority reflected lapses in documentation, not care. Out of 1.46 million reviews completed during the PROs' third contract period, the PROs confirmed 25,724 documentation problems, compared with 6,952 instances of "potential" harm to patients and just 1,116 instances of "actual" harm.

The American Medical Peer Review Association (AMPRA), which lobbies for the PROs in Washington, argues that statistics don't tell the whole story. AMPRA says its members have improved medicine and saved money because of the so-called sentinel effect, a widely acknowledged but hard-to-document phenomenon that prompts physicians and institutions to alter their behavior when they know an authority is watching. Without oversight, AMPRA argues, a number of improvements in care for the elderly might never have come about. The lobbying group maintains that the mere existence of the PRO system has curtailed questionable one-day "observation" stays at hospitals; accelerated the move to outpatient surgery, particularly for cataract extractions; cut down on inappropriate use of assistants in cataract surgery, and helped ensure that cardiac pacemakers are implanted only when they truly benefit patients.

To some extent, review groups probably *have* helped bring about these changes—changes even staunch opponents of government scrutiny generally concede are beneficial. The problem has been that PROs have little or no way of quantifying their contribution. In some areas, common sense suggests they have played a relatively minor role. For instance, the strong financial incentives of the Prospective Payment System (PPS) have surely had a much greater impact on the length of hospital stays than has PRO review. And the trend toward ambulatory surgery was well under way—driven by patient desire and specialty-society endorsement—before PROs began demanding it.

Milwaukee radiologist Thomas Dehn, a former AMPRA president, responds to such comments by citing dramatic changes affecting procedures targeted by the PROs. He claims a "major impact" on the settings in which procedures such as myelograms, cardiac catheterization, and angiography are performed. Before the imposition of PRO review, all these procedures typically required a hospital admission. Today, "it's unusual for us to do them on an inpatient basis," Dr. Dehn says. "We've reversed that 180 degrees."

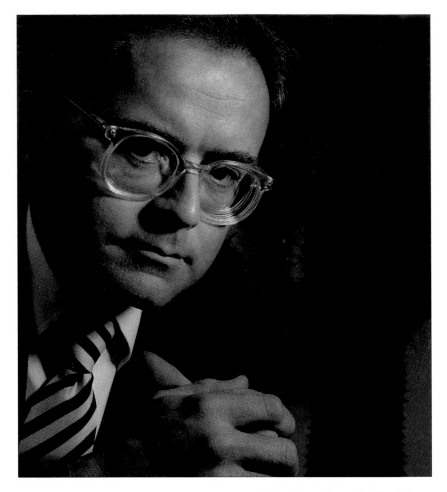

Dr. Thomas Dehn, a former president of the American Medical Peer Review Association (AMPRA), says PROs' falling payment-denial rates show that doctors know they can no longer fool reviewers.

He also contends that preprocedure review, far from being ineffective, has had a big impact on "inefficient physicians who knew they were on thin ice and were willing to change behavior once they were discovered." Preprocedure denial rates—instances in which PROs deny payment for a proposed inpatient procedure—started out high but soon decreased because of "a real quick learning curve," according to Dr. Dehn. In his view, falling denial rates demonstrate the *success* of the review effort, not its failure.

Taking a different tack, some PRO defenders argue that PROs have denied so few requests for elective surgery because HCFA didn't let them go after the admissions most often seen as unnecessary (e.g., admissions for back pain or pneumonia). This contention is supported by findings from the U.S. General Accounting Office (GAO). But the argument usually goes over the heads of those critics who, for all practical purposes, view HCFA and the PROs as one and the same animal.

There's little disagreement that PROs have had an impact in at least one area. "Physicians have made a quantum improvement in their keeping of hospital medical records," says surgeon William Moncrief Jr., the current president of AMPRA and medical director of the California PRO. According to Dr. Moncrief, better documentation translates into better clinical data for outcome studies, and perhaps even better care. "The average practitioner is a little more aware of external oversight," he says, adding that hospitals have responded to review by bolstering internal utilization management and are now "looking hard at every admission."

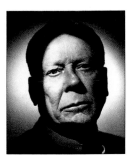

Dr. William Moncrief Jr., the current president of AMPRA.

Dr. Dehn and other PRO advocates also say review has helped counteract the pressures on quality of care brought on by the Prospective Payment System. If DRG-based reimbursement has heightened fears that physicians would discharge patients prematurely to boost hospital revenues, says Dr. Dehn, then PROs have provided "assurance to Medicare beneficiaries that imposition of cost containment hasn't resulted in patterns of compromised care." Radiologist Ira Green, former president of the Virginia PRO, agrees. "Without the PROs, it [pressure to discharge early] would have been a lot worse."

Some outside support for these arguments came in October 1990, when the results of a four-year, $3.9 million Rand Corporation study were published in the *Journal of the American Medical Association*. In one section of the report, researchers analyzed sickness at admission for more than 14,000 Medicare patients admitted to 297 hospitals for five common conditions. The purpose was to compare illness levels before and after the 1983 arrival of PPS. Refuting early speculation that mildly ill people would be admitted more frequently and then quickly discharged to maximize revenue, Rand found that patients were arriving sicker after PPS than before. The authors were tentative in explaining this finding, first suggesting that "better paramedical services" may have helped patients who once would have died en route to a hospital survive long enough to be admitted. But they went on to suggest that financial incentives to hospitals may have been offset by other factors, including peer review.

Finally, anecdotal reports leaked from government agencies suggest that PROs do find and punish a few doctors who are negligent or even dangerous. Though specific grounds for sanctions are generally secret, several horror stories that have escaped suggest how bad patient care occasionally gets.

Consider, for example, a 1986 letter sent by the IG's office to a physician in a Southern state. The letter alleges that the doctor's treatment of one patient included "a failure to make the appropriate diagnosis of myocardial infarction, failure to explore gastrointestinal tract problems, failure of physician to respond in person to changes in patient status when appropriate (after myocardial infarction was recognized), failure to see patient for six hours after admission when appropriate, and premature decision to withdraw life support prior to evidence of irreversible brain damage or brain death." The same physician, in treating another patient, was cited for "failure to recognize and treat congestive heart failure, failure to treat atrial fibrillation with ventricular rate of 120, and failure to prescribe appropriate cardiac medications." For these lapses, the physician got a three-year suspension from Medicare.

Obviously review groups will never please all of their critics, and perhaps won't satisfy any of them. Federal lawmakers tend to be skeptical of the sentinel effect and generally unconcerned about physicians' anger toward the program. They want high "hit" rates to justify a yearly cost of a third of a billion dollars. The IG's office also wants lots of denials and sanction recommendations so it can assure the White House that patient safety and taxpayers' money are being protected. Analysts such as the Institute of Medicine want the program to spend more time looking at trends and patterns of care. Physicians, of course, want PROs to simply go away, or at least operate in a gentle and nonpunitive mode. Any PRO that did so, however, would likely face trouble in its next contract negotiation with HCFA.

CHAPTER TWO

PHYSICIANS VS. THE PROS

For a program so often faulted for having too little effect on the practice of medicine, PROs have generated a remarkable amount of anger among physician groups. Equally remarkable is how quick politicians and government officials have been to lambaste physicians' groups that, despite significant internal problems, have generally made a sincere effort to do the government's bidding. For both sides, peer review has become a symbol. To many physicians, PROs represent decades of federal meddling in the practice of medicine. To the government, the review groups sometimes appear to be all that stands between elderly patients and a horde of health-care providers who would swiftly loot the nation's coffers and perhaps kill a few patients while doing it.

The most celebrated case in the program's history exemplifies the degree of hyperbole surrounding PRO issues. The incident involved New York physician William Diefenbach, whose encounter with the government eventually made national headlines and sparked war between physician groups and federal watchdogs. While the conflict had no obvious heroes or villains, it did illustrate the inherently political nature of governmental quality-assurance efforts and the willingness of all sides to distort facts.

Dr. Diefenbach was by all accounts a kindly small-town physician with deep roots in his community and profession. A general internist who made house calls to his numerous elderly patients, he had enjoyed a quietly successful practice for three decades on the eastern end of New York's Long Island, chiefly in the seaside resorts of Bridgehampton and Southampton.

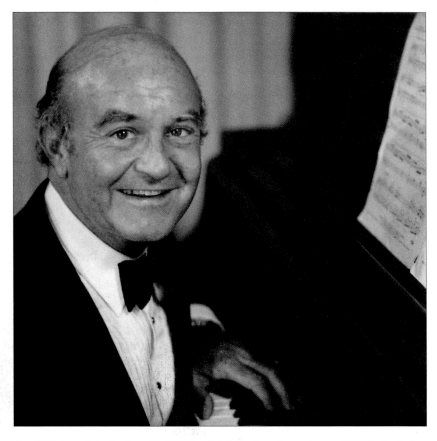

Dr. William Diefenbach's 1990 suicide helped spark an ABC television inquiry into the PRO sanction process. This picture was taken in 1986, the same year he was suspended from Medicare.

Then, in the mid-1980s, the New York State peer review organization began scrutinizing his work; routine review had signaled problems with the care of some of his patients. The PRO investigation eventually found evidence that Dr. Diefenbach had "grossly and flagrantly" violated quality-of-care standards in treating five Medicare and four Medicaid patients at Southampton Hospital. In August 1986, the review group recommended to the HHS inspector general that Dr. Diefenbach, 63, be barred from the Medicare program. Forever.

The IG's office, after weighing the evidence, handed down a reduced sentence: Dr. Diefenbach would be suspended from Medicare for five years. He received the news of his punishment shortly before Christmas 1986 in a letter from the IG's sanctions chief,

A Shift in Perspective ...

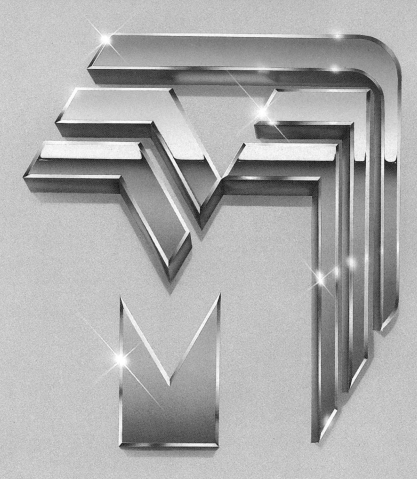

The flexibility to shift perspective is key to creativity and innovation. Sometimes a closer view or a different angle reveals a whole new truth. Sometimes it takes a step back to see the larger picture. At Marion Merrell Dow we are committed to an ongoing effort to discover, explore, and deal with reality by looking at our world from various and differing points of view.

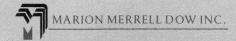

MARION MERRELL DOW INC.

James Patton. Patton's letter offered few clinical details. But it did say that Dr. Diefenbach had ordered "multiple medications without waiting to determine their effect." The IG's office backed the PRO in all nine cases. It found Dr. Diefenbach guilty of, as the letter put it, "one or more instances which present an imminent danger to the health, safety, or well-being of a Medicare beneficiary or place the beneficiary unnecessarily in high-risk situations."

Patton's letter also zeroed in on inconsistencies between Dr. Diefenbach's documentation and his subsequent explanations of treatment. Patton wrote that "either the patient was ill as the medical chart suggests, and the care you provided did not meet professionally recognized standards, or, if your response is credited, and the patient's diagnosis and the progress notes were not accurate, then the patient's admission to the hospital was not necessary." He had a point. Dr. Diefenbach's records apparently suggested a pattern of inadequate care for seriously ill patients. His subsequent testimony implied that the patients had been too healthy to admit to a hospital. Meanwhile, the fact that a patient had died seemed to back the records. Either way, Patton saw little hope of rehabilitation. The letter said that although Dr. Diefenbach seemed willing to improve, he appeared unable to do so.

Dr. Diefenbach exercised his legal right to request a hearing on the expulsion before a federal administrative law judge in February 1987. But before the hearing could take place, he entered into settlement discussions with the IG's office. By fall, a proposed settlement had been sent to the physician's attorney. Details of the proposed deal have never been revealed, but presumably it offered something less than the five-year sentence. Oddly, though, Dr. Diefenbach never signed it. Nor did he request intervention from the administrative law judge. Instead, he simply allowed the five-year sentence to take effect.

In June 1990, three and a half years into his sentence, Dr. Diefenbach put a pistol to his head and pulled the trigger.

The controversy might have been buried along with Dr. Diefenbach had it not been for ABC television reporter Chris Wallace, who resurrected the Diefenbach case in September 1990 during a *PrimeTime Live* segment on questionable tactics used by government investigators of health-care fraud. In the piece, Dr. Diefenbach's patient care was staunchly defended by Dr. Robert Fear, then the medical-staff president of Southampton Hospital, who recalled being "amazed" when he'd heard his colleague was the subject of a federal quality-of-care investigation. "They couldn't possibly be

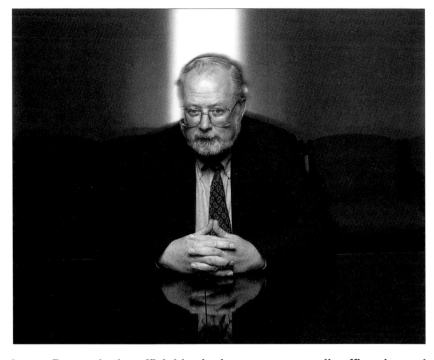

James Patton is the official in the inspector general's office charged with deciding whether to uphold or modify a PRO's recommendation to suspend or expel a physician from Medicare.

talking about Bill Diefenbach," he remembered thinking.

Wallace presented other information that seemed to cast doubt on the government's charges. A hospital investigation prompted by the PRO's allegations had turned up poor record-keeping but no evidence of harm to patients. Dr. Diefenbach's wife protested on camera that the IG had not bothered to interview her husband's patients. And Dr. Diefenbach himself offered a defense of his care via footage from a 1987 television interview. He calmly explained that he'd been targeted for lack of documentation. "I didn't write enough on my charts, and I admit that," he said. "I spent most of my time with my patients, with their families."

To tell the government's side, Wallace chose HHS inspector general Richard Kusserow, a former FBI and CIA agent who had a history of skirmishes with organized medicine. In an interview, Wallace pressed Kusserow for evidence that Diefenbach's transgressions involved more than documentation, and got a stunning response.

Kusserow: There was evidence in a number of cases that he was an impaired physician, he was suffering from drug abuse, and as a result of that, he was considered unwilling or unable to change. . . .

Wallace: Drug abuse?

Kusserow: Yes.

Wallace: Where? I mean, I must say he was never charged with that.

Kusserow: This person was providing second-class medicine. He did not belong in the program.

Wallace: We will go back and check, and if there's evidence of drug abuse, that's . . . something that we absolutely were unaware of.

Kusserow: You can jam it down my throat [if I'm wrong]. Jam it down my throat.

Wallace was happy to oblige. He went back to the senior physician at Southampton Hospital, who proclaimed there wasn't "a shred of evidence" Dr. Diefenbach had abused drugs. And the physician's widow seemed dumbfounded by the new allegations.

Mrs. Diefenbach: Are you serious? He said that? That man is . . . it's a total, complete, utter, devastating lie. He had better have proof of that.

As it turned out, there was no proof. A week later, before the program was aired, Kusserow issued a carefully worded statement in which he defended the Medicare expulsion but retracted the drug charge. The normally combative IG declined to appear on camera this time and asked journalists to drop the matter. Instead, ABC aired the accusation and then the text of the retraction.

The IG's office began trying to minimize the damage. Reporters were told Kusserow had been misled by a staffer during a prebroadcast strategy meeting. Kusserow's press office called ABC's piece a "hatchet job." And the IG went to unusual lengths to show that even without drug charges, Dr. Diefenbach's expulsion had been justified. One statement from Kusserow's office noted that some 30 physicians had had a hand in reviewing the nine cases. Another statement outlined the clinical issues. What the IG acted on, it said, were PRO findings that Dr. Diefenbach had "mishandled heart-condition patients by not ordering necessary tests, failing to recognize and treat serious heart conditions, and furnishing multiple medications without considering their possible effect on the patients." Sanctions chief Patton reminded the press that it was Dr. Diefenbach who had opted not to accept a negotiated settlement, and that years separated the sanction and suicide.

The American Medical Association, however, lost no time demanding the IG's immediate ouster for once again having trampled physicians' rights. Kusserow's gaffe was just another example of his penchant for "reckless and unfounded charges," the group asserted.

In a letter to President Bush, Dr. Joseph T. Painter, chairman of the AMA board of trustees, proclaimed that "whatever else he may assert about his record, Mr. Kusserow can no longer claim to have the trust of the medical profession and our patients."

The AMA used several means to keep the embarrassing story in the headlines. The group invited reporters to its Washington office to view the ABC videotape, and staffers circulated copies on Capitol Hill. AMA officials also used the Diefenbach episode to revive earlier criticisms of the IG, including the charge that targeted physicians were deprived of due process. The AMA said it wanted a new IG

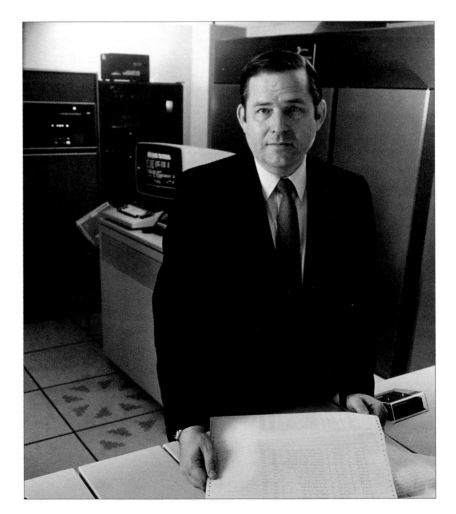

Richard Kusserow, inspector general of Health and Human Services, retracted his allegation that Dr. Diefenbach had abused drugs but defended his office's decision to penalize the doctor.

who wasn't involved in a vendetta against the medical profession. After only a week, the group was boasting that its chances of getting rid of the IG were "better than fifty-fifty." But in early 1991, months after the AMA's initial call to arms, the IG remained in power, backed publicly by HHS secretary Dr. Louis Sullivan.

To hear the AMA tell it, the Diefenbach incident was straightforward. A doctor no longer in a position to defend himself had been wrongly accused of drug abuse on national television by an irresponsible federal official who couldn't get his facts straight and then refused to apologize. It was one more example of an overzealous federal gumshoe trampling the rights of a defenseless doctor. And the AMA implied that not only had Kusserow's comments been wrong, but the entire PRO case against Diefenbach probably amounted to little more than evidence of shoddy paperwork— another example of irresponsible scalp-hunting by a review group.

But the AMA's version of the affair left out some important elements. One was that the recommendation to exclude Dr. Diefenbach came only after exhaustive review by an extremely cautious PRO, the Empire State Medical, Scientific and Educational Foundation of Lake Success. Because the charges concerned many patients, literally dozens of physicians were involved in the review process, making bias or misinterpretation unlikely. Also, the initial recommendation to sanction Dr. Diefenbach had come from a review group that was a subcontractor to the New York PRO. As a result, the evidence and recommendations were reexamined by the PRO's own board of directors before being submitted to the government. This meant an extra layer of review before the case even reached the IG's office.

In addition, the AMA didn't mention that the New York PRO was a creation of the state medical society and had a national reputation for lenience. Started by the Medical Society of the State of New York, Empire held the PRO contract from 1984 to 1989. The group was frequently criticized for inaction by consumer groups, the IG's office, HCFA, and even its subcontractors. Critics said the PRO rarely bothered to follow up its own findings of poor care. During the six years Empire held the PRO contract, they noted, only two physicians were sanctioned. One was Dr. Diefenbach.

Confidential memoranda from HCFA to the PRO in the late 1980s blasted Empire for shoddy record-keeping, lax internal management systems, and repeated failure to act quickly against physicians found to be providing substandard care. Amid much rancor, the PRO was replaced by one of its former subcontractors, a Long Island-based physicians' organization, in December 1989. In this context, Empire's recommendation not only to punish Dr. Diefenbach but also to expel him permanently takes on special meaning. Even aggressive PROs usually favor punishments of five years or less for all but the most blatant offenders.

Also absent from the AMA version was the fact that Kusserow's office reduced Dr. Diefenbach's punishment from life to five years and that the IG's office had reviewed the findings of both the PRO and its subcontractor. In his letter to Dr. Diefenbach, Patton stated that before acting he had carefully reviewed the evidence, including the hospital's own investigation. Kusserow may have botched his interview with ABC, but there was no sign his case against Dr. Diefenbach was biased or tainted.

Finally, in its revived assault on the PRO program in general, the AMA did not mention its own links with the review group that brought down Dr. Diefenbach. As one of a handful of PROs sponsored by a state medical society, Empire had the AMA's tacit blessing and support. The AMA has urged medical societies to form PROs, possibly as a way to keep disciplinary responsibilities out of less sympathetic hands. And it has offered support to these presumably friendly PROs in the form of workshops and conferences on at least two occasions.

Taken as a whole, the Diefenbach case provides a window on the highly politicized world of government regulation of health-care quality, revealing both strengths and flaws in the process. The system includes more than its share of red tape and at least one federal official who appears to take lightly the effect a disciplinary action or casual remark can have on a physician's life, career, and reputation. But the peer review program also provides physicians with substantial protection from capricious actions by reviewers or government officials. Charges can be appealed at several levels, and before imposing a severe sanction the government must deem a physician not only guilty of infractions but also unwilling or unable to change. Moreover, the Diefenbach episode shows that although doctors may be questioned about clinical decisions, they rarely face disciplinary action. In one of the nation's most populous states, sanctions were handed out to just two doctors in five years. For at least one of them it took nine separate incidents, dozens of review doctors, and an investigation that spanned years before his right to treat Medicare patients was contested.

CHAPTER THREE

BUILDING THE PROS

I n theory, PROs are steady, vigilant guardians of patients and the Medicare trust fund. In practice, they are unpredictable, driven by business motives as much as a desire to protect the public, and often unsure whether to play the role of policeman or educator. Moreover, the PROs are forever trying to balance the desires of a tightfisted Congress, a prescriptive bureaucracy, and a perpetually enraged physician population. If PROs' actions seem confusing, that is partly because of the contradictory forces that propel them and the competing masters they serve.

Of course, the PROs didn't achieve their present state overnight. It took years and the concerted efforts of a slew of individuals and groups.

Peer review organizations were created by Congress in 1982 to replace the equally controversial professional standards review organizations. PSROs had been mandated a decade earlier to ensure high-quality care and to check rapidly rising Medicare hospital costs. It is widely agreed they did neither. PSROs established a reputation as torpid watchdogs, lacking the authority and, in many cases, the desire to question doctors' decisions. So, Congress decided to start afresh. The new guardians, lawmakers vowed, would have real clout and would be held accountable for specific objectives, such as reducing nosocomial infection rates.

The 195 nonprofit PSROs, which had operated under noncompetitive annual grants that had imposed few explicit objectives, were consolidated into 54 PROs, most defined by state boundaries, and all were assigned to one of 10 regional operating offices. They would operate under two-year fixed-price contracts decided by competitive bidding. It was made clear that PROs that failed to perform would lose their contracts to more capable competitors.

Bidders could be not-for-profit or for-profit entities, as long as they were either run by doctors or able to show they could recruit local physicians willing to do peer review. Groups run by doctors were to be given preference. Although the law allowed out-of-state bids, Congress favored local entities. Lawmakers reasoned that in-state groups would be better accepted by county medical societies and couldn't be viewed as medical carpetbaggers out to earn a few bucks by slashing away at some other state's expenditures.

Unlike PSROs, PROs would get all of their contract money directly from the Medicare trust funds—a provision intended to shield them from the vagaries of Congress's annual appropriations process. PROs would also be given highly specific (some said prescriptive) objectives. And the new organizations wouldn't be allowed, as the old ones had been, to delegate review duties to the very hospitals that were being reviewed.

Nonetheless, PROs resembled their defunct cousins in some important ways. Like PSROs, PROs were given the authority to review medical records and deny hospital payments. Similarly, PROs could recommend that substandard physicians and hospitals be fined or expelled from Medicare. Review experts said this sanction authority, though not popular with doctors, was the only sure way to get the attention of recalcitrant physicians and institutions. (The authority was strengthened significantly by a provision stating that if the inspector general failed to rule on a case promptly, the sanctions recommended by a PRO would be implemented until the IG did rule.) A final similarity was the staffs. Many PSRO executives found new homes at PROs, and a good many physicians who had served on PSRO boards became PRO directors.

In a move designed to attract support from organized medicine, state medical societies were permitted to sponsor PROs. A handful of society-sponsored review groups (Massachusetts', for example) are still in operation. Medical society involvement in peer review, however, hasn't prevented the American Medical Association from blasting the whole program regularly at its meetings. To bolster PROs' private-sector credentials, the new groups were encouraged to accept outside review work. Today, most have contracts to perform reviews for CHAMPUS, the Defense Department's civilian health program. And many work for state Medicaid agencies. A

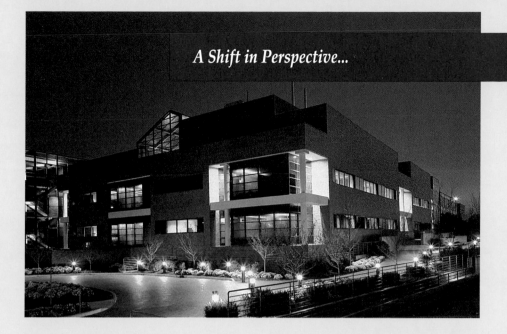

A Shift in Perspective...

Work Locally...

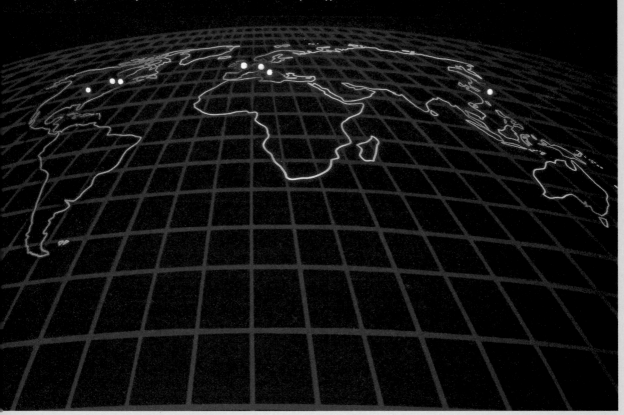

A Shift in Perspective Makes a World of Difference

Work Locally but Think Globally

Around the world, Marion Merrell Dow research centers are home to hundreds
of physicians and scientists whose curiosity and joy of discovery are nurtured
in an atmosphere of freedom, openness, and informality. In Cincinnati, Kansas
City, and Indianapolis...in Strasbourg, France and Gerenzano, Italy...in
Winnersh, England and Hirakata, Japan—local Marion Merrell Dow associates
look for innovative approaches and new perspectives in pharmacology.
At each local facility, the view is global.

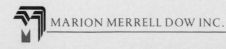

MARION MERRELL DOW INC.

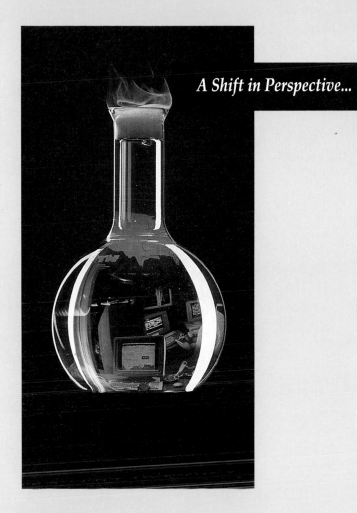

Beyond Science and Technology...

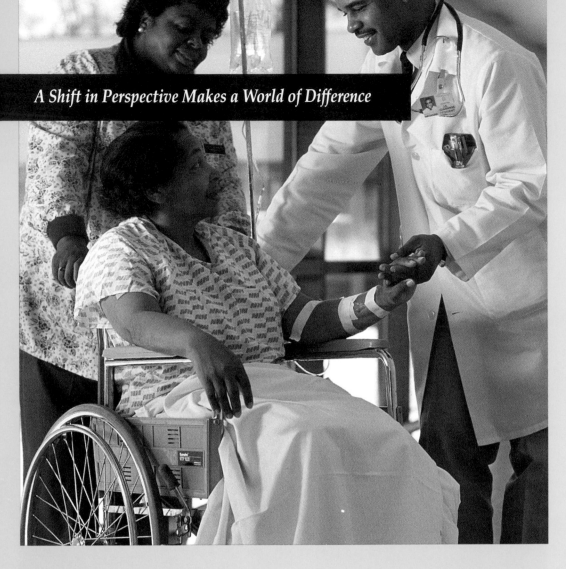

A Shift in Perspective Makes a World of Difference

Beyond Science and Technology...
Our Vision Is of Humanity

Wherever our research takes us, we never lose sight of its ultimate goal—
improving the human condition. Alleviating pain and suffering. Improving the
quality of life. Enabling the disabled. Extending the span of health and vigor.
When we look at a molecule, with a shift in perspective, we see a human being.

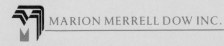

MARION MERRELL DOW INC.

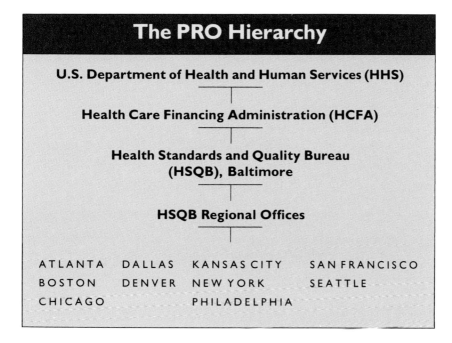

The PRO Hierarchy

U.S. Department of Health and Human Services (HHS)

Health Care Financing Administration (HCFA)

**Health Standards and Quality Bureau
(HSQB), Baltimore**

HSQB Regional Offices

ATLANTA	DALLAS	KANSAS CITY	SAN FRANCISCO
BOSTON	DENVER	NEW YORK	SEATTLE
CHICAGO		PHILADELPHIA	

few have substantial contracts with private insurers.

But the PROs' bread and butter remains Medicare review, and their major employer is the Health Care Financing Administration. The program is managed nationally by career bureaucrats in a division of HCFA known as the Health Standards and Quality Bureau (HSQB). HCFA's central office is a fortresslike structure in Baltimore enclosing a maze of corridors and thousands of staffers who control more than $100 billion in health-care spending each year. Day-to-day responsibilities, however, are shouldered by officials in the regional offices.

The key federal officials dealing with the PROs are generally not physicians. Acting on PRO sanction recommendations, for example, is the responsibility of HHS inspector general Kusserow, who serves at the pleasure of the president. Sanctions chief Patton is likewise a career health-care official without medical credentials. For advice on clinical matters, Patton keeps full-time physicians on staff and also consults doctors at Walter Reed Army Hospital, among others, for second opinions on specific sanction cases.

Since the PRO program's inception, Congress has rarely resisted the impulse to tinker with it. Changes generally arrive in the late fall or winter as obscure amendments buried within the massive annual federal budget bill. These modifications have affected PRO funding, review areas, jurisdiction, and bidding procedures. Often the alterations smack of pressure from interest groups—a 1990 provision, for instance, specifies that PROs try to use podiatrists rather than M.D.'s or D.O.'s to review podiatric cases. Overall, Congress has been moving the program away from its initial preoccupation with hospital costs toward an emphasis on quality of care in a variety of health-care settings—a move plagued with difficulties even by PRO standards.

Ironically, this push for quality reflects federal efforts at cost cutting. With the advent of the Prospective Payment System in 1983—a program that gave hospitals financial incentives strong enough to chop inpatient stays by 20 percent—lawmakers worried that patient care might be at risk. They feared that greedy hospitals would urge doctors to discharge patients prematurely or transfer them inappropriately from beds covered by PPS to psychiatric or other beds still reimbursed under the old system. Lawmakers also wondered whether an epidemic of very brief admissions of comparatively healthy patients would ensue. No elected official wanted to be the one trying to explain on television why the government, in its quest for efficiency, hadn't taken steps to ensure that Aunt Bess got the care she deserved.

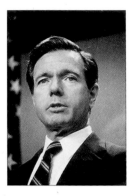

Senator John Heinz charged PPS caused patients to be released "quicker and sicker."

Senator John Heinz, a Pennsylvania Republican who has never been described as camera-shy, quickly embraced the issue, alleging that hospitals were discharging patients "quicker and sicker." His anecdotal horror stories have since been largely discredited by statistical studies. The Massachusetts-based Health Data Institute, for instance, found evidence of premature discharge in only 1.1 percent of more than 7,000 records from 1984 and 1985. And, as noted, a $3.9 million Rand Corporation study of more than 14,000 records from 297 hospitals found fewer instances of poor-quality Medicare inpatient services after PPS than before.

But such studies hadn't yet appeared when Congress named PROs as the force that would protect elderly patients from the dark side of reimbursement reform. To make sure the groups really could guard senior citizens, lawmakers sharpened review of discharge planning, transfers, and readmissions. Congress also enacted legislation to prevent hospitals from transferring slow-healing patients to nursing facilities and home health agencies. But these were merely stopgap measures. The new rules of hospital payment, coupled with technological advances, guaranteed that more and more care would be provided outside of hospitals. If the government was going to monitor treatment, it would have to loose its watchdogs on outpatient facilities, HMOs, and perhaps even physicians' offices.

Slowly, painfully, the move to extend the scope of PROs beyond inpatient review is taking place. By spring 1989, all PROs had the authority to review Medicare patient records not only in hospitals but also in HMOs, skilled nursing facilities, home health agencies, hospital outpatient departments, and ambulatory-surgery centers. Review of HMO services was sporadic through 1990, though, because of persistent problems review groups experienced in trying to obtain inpatient medical records of Medicare beneficiaries enrolled in the prepaid plans. Also, HCFA chose to limit review of skilled nursing facilities and home health agencies to a relatively small number of "intervening care" cases, in which a patient discharged from a hospital is readmitted within 31 days. Review of ambulatory-surgery centers likewise has been minimal.

In 1990, the Wisconsin and Maryland PROs were awarded contracts for pilot review of Medicare services provided in physicians' private offices, a step that many physicians see as the ultimate threat to their autonomy.

The steady expansion of review has helped many PROs become thriving businesses. Total federal spending on the PROs' third set of contracts, which runs from 1988 to 1991, comes to nearly $1 billion. PRO contracts range from a high of $82.8 million in California to $1.2 million in Wyoming. But HCFA has offset some of the cost of expanded review by requiring review of fewer records in each category. At one time, PROs were reviewing nearly half of all Medicare hospitalizations. That rate fell to less than 20 percent in 1990 and was expected to fall to 10 percent in 1991.

If the government continues to ask PROs to review fewer records in more care settings, critics will undoubtedly ask whether the effort has been emasculated. But for physicians, the change could provide relief from frequent questioning. Already the chance of a given Medicare hospital admission's being reviewed is just one in five. As that figure falls to one in 10, doctors can expect fewer letters from PROs and fewer payment denials.

CHAPTER FOUR

THE POLICYMAKERS

T here's nothing glamorous about the life of a PRO employee. Review nurses spend their days combing stacks of illegible or nearly illegible medical charts in central offices or in cramped hospital record rooms. Medical-records technicians face an even drearier routine: they spend all day checking records to ensure that DRG codes are accurate. And, though a PRO's board of directors may include leading physicians, its physician-advisers—paid $50 to $80 an hour to sift through charts—are rarely prominent. Many review doctors are young; many are also loners with idealistic views about medicine's need to police itself. A large part of their job consists of taking angry phone calls from attendings who challenge the reviewing physician's credentials. It's tedious, punishing work.

In fact, the only place where the quality-assurance business gets really interesting is in Washington, D.C. There, life crackles with excitement for the phalanx of lobbyists, attorneys, consultants, bureaucrats, medical directors, and think-tank specialists involved in setting PRO policy. Few have ever been within spitting distance of a medical-records room. The daily routine for these people includes composing position papers and negotiating with the power brokers in Congress. The PRO world's movers and shakers are versed in political infighting and know how to start a rumor without leaving footprints. Some even enjoy a limited celebrity: PRO policy heavyweights include people with nicknames like General Patton and the Junkyard Dog. But flamboyance aside, they embody the values and set the tone for a program that affects the daily life of nearly every physician in America.

At the top of the PRO heap is a troika of administrators whose names are familiar to many physicians. Thomas Morford, director of the Health Standards and Quality Bureau, has overall management responsibility for the 54 PROs, shared authority with 10 regional HCFA offices, and direct control of a staff of about 90 that works exclusively on the program in Baltimore. The office of Richard Kusserow, inspector general of the Department of Health and Human Services, decides whether to approve PRO sanction recommendations. Health Care Financing adminstrator Gail Wilensky is Morford's boss, and she is responsible for overseeing a myriad of other policy proposals like physician payment reform, enhanced clinical laboratory oversight, and the revamping of the way hospital capital costs are reimbursed. But when PROs are in the news, Morford and Kusserow most often make the headlines.

Morford took over as director of HSQB in the summer of 1986. A born bureaucrat, he has a knack for public speeches that are substantive yet general enough not to irk pressure groups. His current position isn't a political appointment, but that's a long way from saying it isn't political. Congressmen call him when a favored review group loses its contract. PRO lobbyists call him when they object to a new federal requirement. Medical societies call him to threaten lawsuits over local review disputes. And PRO executives call him to complain about the bureaucrats in regional offices.

A career health-care official with a calm exterior that conceals a strong temper, Morford isn't given to rash or emotional decisions. He is credited with stabilizing the program, introducing objective management controls, and emphasizing continuity. During his tenure as chief, only a handful of PROs have been forced to compete to renew their contracts, and every contested contract decision has been backed by the General Accounting Office. A skillful infighter when dealing with the Office of Management and Budget and Congress, Morford takes credit for increasing PRO funding, developing staggered, less frantic three-year contract cycles, and introducing a point system (the Quality Intervention Plan, or QIP) for keeping track of physician quality-of-care demerits. He is also the power behind the Uniform Clinical Data Set (UCDS), a system that requires PROs to record a standard set of clinical information for each case they review.

Morford has fared considerably better as director than his predecessor, Philip Nathanson, who weathered four years in the job

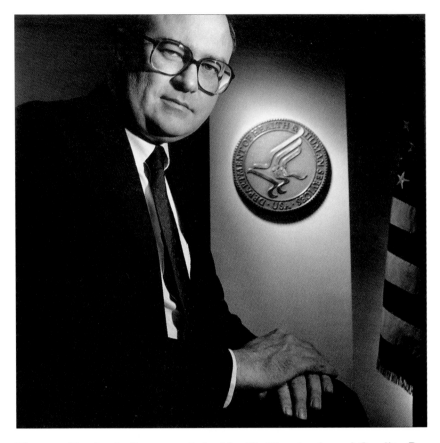

Thomas Morford, director of the Health Standards and Quality Bureau, is credited with stabilizing federal supervision of the PROs.

before resigning to take a hospital quality-assurance post in California in 1986. Nathanson is best remembered for his decision the same year to put up for competitive bid roughly half of all existing PRO contracts because he felt the groups were not performing well. Though most PRO contractors ultimately retained their franchises, that bloodletting, just two years into the first contract, led both lobbyists and PROs to accuse Nathanson of playing favorites and threatening groups that publicly criticized him—charges he strongly denies.

The current director likes to refer to the dangers of "whipsawing the program because someone got a bright idea." His approach to change is usually incremental, with lobbying groups assured they'll be heard before anything of consequence happens. A leader who guards his program jealously against attempts to expand it willynilly, Morford is hostile to congressionally mandated forays into review of HMOs, skilled nursing facilities, and home health agencies. His goal is to establish PROs as credible reviewers of inpatient care before permitting wholesale expansion into nonhospital settings. He is candid about deficiencies in his agency's performance and appears to have no illusions about the analytic capabilities of some of the regional office personnel with whom he shares program-management responsibilities.

The most frequent criticism of the HSQB chief is that he's overworked, has spread himself dangerously thin, and is at the mercy of an uneven staff. In addition to managing the PRO program, Morford is in charge of the federal health-care survey and certification system, which regulates everything from hospitals and nursing homes to home health agencies and clinical labs. If that weren't enough, he's also the point man for HCFA's annual public release of institution-specific Medicare mortality data on about 6,000 American hospitals, an event that enrages physician and hospital groups that claim the data is of little relevance. Political heat from the mortality data alone might have felled a lesser man, and some view it as a factor in Nathanson's resignation.

Morford's sole professional passion seems to be the Uniform Clinical Data Set. This ambitious project is an attempt to automate and standardize initial PRO screenings using computerized algorithms, which will create a massive clinical database. The data are to be used for clinical outcomes research and could play a major role in the development of practice parameters for physicians. Morford's determination to complete the project is intense and undisguised. In the autumn of 1990, in a rare baring of teeth, he told a meeting of PRO officials in Chicago that they would begin automating initial case screenings if he had to drag them all kicking and screaming to do it. "If any of you don't believe that you can do it, believe that I have will enough for both of us," he said.

The federal official most often at odds with Morford and HSQB is HHS inspector general Kusserow. Unlike Morford, Kusserow is known as something of a buccaneer and showman who makes little effort to hide a Broadway-sized taste for headlines. A career law-enforcement official, he was nominated to his position by Ronald Reagan in 1981 and reappointed by George Bush in 1990. Kusserow had 13 years of experience with the FBI, for which he worked against organized crime in Chicago. Before that he was with the CIA, in a position he declines to describe. Tagged as the quintessential "junkyard dog" by his admirers in Congress and elsewhere, he is heavy-set, blunt, and widely perceived as crude. Kusserow once told a gathering of PRO representatives that the problem with administrative law judges, who often reverse his Medicare exclusions, is that many are "brain-dead."

Considerably higher than Morford in the HHS pecking order, Kusserow is appointed by the president and can't be replaced even by the secretary of HHS. Therefore, he sees himself as a goad to the federal bureaucracy. The inspector general's office produces blizzards of quickie analyses, cost estimates, and management reports. These often draw criticism on methodological grounds and almost invariably embarrass HSQB.

Kusserow's influence on the PRO program comes largely from his ability to set its tone despite limited involvement in the review process. The IG's only direct responsibility to the PROs lies in deciding whether or not to approve recommended disciplinary actions against physicians, a duty that has been fully delegated to sanctions chief James Patton. Kusserow has never been accused of interfering with Patton's decisions. But the IG has sent letters to PROs reminding them of their obligation to refer cases worthy of sanction—letters the AMA has characterized as pressure tactics.

If not for Patton, Kusserow might well be under heavier fire. Though some in HCFA refer to him as "General Patton" because of his punctilious adherence to statutory requirements, he is a cordial, self-effacing career official. Patton makes no excuses for turning down roughly 40 percent of the sanction recommendations PROs send him, and he's a demon for due process and the letter of the law. His methods belie the notion that Kusserow's staff runs roughshod over physicians.

Bush appointee Gail Wilensky's nomination as HCFA administrator was confirmed by the Senate in February 1990. An economist by training, Wilensky was vice-president of Project Hope, where she concentrated on the problems of health insurance for the uninsured. Her job is extremely demanding; in fact, most of her predecessors have lasted no more than three or four years. Almost from the moment she started work, for example, she came under pressure from the Group Health Association of America, which strongly opposes PRO review of HMOs. The GHAA persuaded the new administrator to order her staff to develop strategies that would let reviewers place more emphasis on HMOs' own internal quality-assurance systems, as opposed to PRO guidelines. Months later, Wilensky, who had been a champion of managed care, admitted that she had ordered the proposed changes without seeing statistical results on HMO quality performance under the existing review

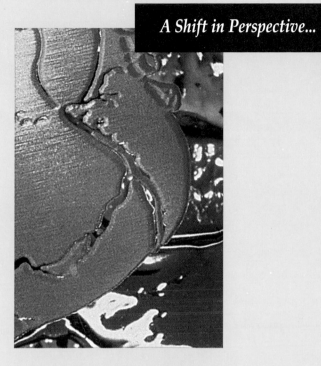

Behind Every Cardizem and Cardizem SR Prescription...

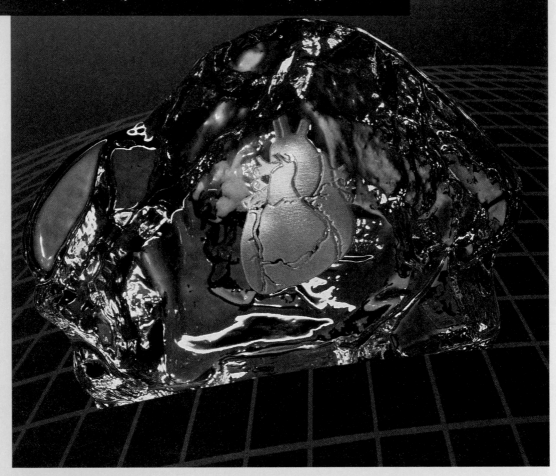
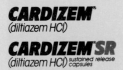
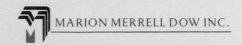

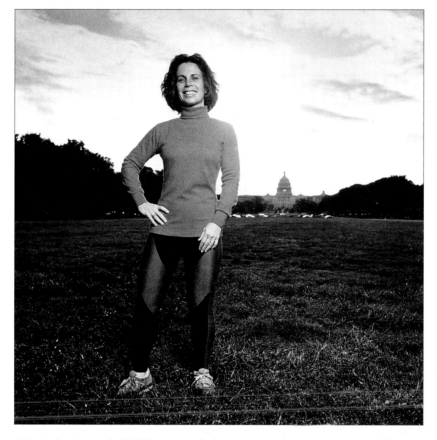

**Administrator Gail Wilensky of the Health Care Financing Adminis-
tration backs Morford's plan for the Uniform Clinical Data Set.**

system. Still in draft form, the final revised plan was scheduled for
release in early 1991.

The most rancorous battle of Wilensky's tenure so far, however,
is not about PROs but about Medicare Part B review in Georgia. By
1990, many Georgia physicians had become incensed about the
performance and methods of HealthCare Compare, an Illinois-
based utilization-review firm hired by Aetna, Georgia's Part B carrier, to scrutinize office-based expenditures. In the face of physician
protests, Wilensky renewed HealthCare Compare's funding, and
doctors charged that political cronyism had influenced her decision. They have threatened to sue both Wilensky and her agency.

In the PRO arena, Wilensky has so far followed Morford's recommendations. She supports his UCDS plan, which she sees as a means
of emphasizing health-care outcomes analysis, thereby redirecting
the PRO program from prescriptive rulemaking to marshaling facts

to build consensus about the most effective treatment plans.

Counterbalancing these three government administrators are entities that represent consumers, physicians, and advocacy groups. Though their agendas vary widely, each has left a mark on thc program. The groups that exert the most influence over PROs' day-to-day operations are the tiny American Medical Peer Review Association (AMPRA); the elephantine American Association of Retired Persons (AARP); the AMA; and the American Hospital Association (AHA).

AMPRA, the PROs' own lobby, is run by a youthful and energetic staff whose members are on a first-name basis with all the important agency and Capitol Hill staffers. Its pair of 30-something leaders are executive vice-president Andrew Webber and associate executive vice-president Lisa Looper. He is an immaculate, blow-dried Harvard graduate who gets high marks for performance. She is a savvy lobbyist who worked her way up from the secretarial pool.

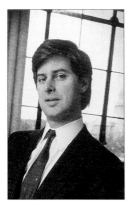

Andrew Webber is AMPRA's executive vice-president.

Often underestimated by the competition, AMPRA consistently succeeds in sponsoring small but significant legislative changes that get slipped into last-minute federal budget reconciliation acts. A case in point was the inclusion in the 1990 budget of technical language that extends civil and criminal immunity to PROs as corporate entities. The young staff avoids confrontation and is careful to defer major policy questions to senior physician leaders. AMPRA's current president is Dr. William Moncrief Jr., a thoracic and vascular surgeon.

The AMA has long functioned as the PROs' chief nemesis, leading the fight against what it views as the program's lack of due-process safeguards for the physicians it targets. And the physicians' group has had some successes: following the filing of a suit in federal court in 1987, HHS agreed to permit physicians' attorneys to be present at meetings before formal recommendations to sanction; to provide prompt access to verbatim transcripts of meetings; and to exclude the PRO physicians who originally investigated a doctor from voting on whether to recommend a sanction. Lately, however, there has been talk of establishing better lines of communication between the PROs and the AMA, probably because of the 1990 elevation of Dr. James Todd to the position of AMA executive vice-president. Dr. Todd told members gathered at the House of Delegates meeting in Orlando in December 1990 that "the politics of confrontation are no longer suitable as they were in the past."

Throughout the 1980s, the AMA's policy on PROs was the personal province of Dr. James Sammons, a Texan with loads of good-old-boy charm who became a bare-knuckles combatant at any hint of transgression against his membership. In 1990, Dr. Sammons retired early from the top AMA staff job amid accusations of financial impropriety. Dr. Todd is viewed as something of a technocrat in comparison with Dr. Sammons.

Dr. Todd has observer status at AMPRA's thrice-yearly board meetings, and he has told the PRO lobbying group he intends to continue attending in person. He also supports the aims of Dr. John Kelly, a former California PRO executive, who is the cautious director of the newly created AMA Office of Quality Assurance. The appointment of Dr. Kelly was considered shrewd, since the AMA's commitment to quality assurance had long been in question. Previously, the group had been accused of playing to the crowd at its House of Delegates meetings by having its leaders speak in favor of quality measures in general while delegates routinely voted down specific mechanisms for change.

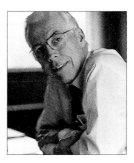

Dr. James Todd became executive vice-president of the AMA in 1990.

Dr. Kelly's challenge is to help the AMA do more than just shout down outsiders' proposals. To this end, the group has begun working with the Rand Corporation and academic centers to develop practice guidelines for physicians. But some still doubt the AMA's commitment. Veteran AMA-basher Fortney "Pete" Stark (D-Calif.), who chairs the subcommittee on health of the House Ways and Means Committee, pointed out to Dr. Kelly in a 1989 get-acquainted hearing that the budget for Dr. Kelly's entire quality-assurance division at the time was roughly equal to Dr. Sammons' annual pay package—about $700,000 by the time he retired last year.

The American Association of Retired Persons, whose 32.5 million members make it potentially the most formidable lobby in Washington, is something of a disappointment to allies and even to some of its own staff. Since losing a couple of head-to-head battles with the AMA over PRO sanction authority in 1987, the group has seemed increasingly tentative. AARP suffered its biggest public humiliation the following year when Medicare catastrophic-coverage legislation, which it had endorsed, prompted massive protests from its members. Congress repealed catastrophic coverage in 1989, and a few lawmakers accused AARP of being out of touch with its members. Lately the group has focused on encouraging the exchange of information between PROs and state licensing boards. And it continues to lobby quietly for legislation that would better define PROs' authority to determine which substandard physicians are "willing or able" to improve. The group also continues to fund a

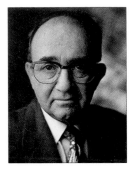

Dr. James Sammons led the AMA during the last decade.

consumer-outreach program that offers education and technical assistance to consumer members on PRO boards. Critics argue that the group's inability to target a few PRO issues and hammer away at them, combined with a reluctance to make political enemies, has sharply limited its ability to affect the program at all.

The American Hospital Association has a seat at the monthly meeting Morford holds for provider and consumer representatives, but AHA seems to devote fewer resources to PRO legislation than other groups do. That's not to say the AHA doesn't get exercised from time to time: since the late 1980s, it's been fighting a rancorous and seemingly endless legal battle with HHS over reimbursement for PRO-requested photocopies of medical records. AHA wants 12 cents a page for photocopying; HHS currently. provides a nickel. Though it's a battle worth millions if it ever gets resolved, it's not the sort of issue that excites anyone other than the attorneys involved. (Technically, AHA's fight has been subsumed into a national class-action suit on behalf of its member hospitals.)

A fifth group that sometimes figures in conflicts over PRO issues is the Joint Commission on Accreditation of Healthcare Organizations (JCAHO), headed by Dr. Dennis O'Leary. Under Dr. O'Leary, JCAHO has gone up against the PROs for control of the Medicare quality-assurance agenda, seeking to move the feds away from regulation and toward voluntarism and clinical-consensus building. Because JCAHO is in the quality-assurance business itself, a shift in this direction could mean a larger role for the organization in quality oversight. Thus Dr. O'Leary's frequent quips at the expense of the PRO program, always delivered elegantly. When PROs replaced the professional standards review organizations, he was quick to tag them "PSROs without the standards."

While the interplay between HCFA, HSQB, the IG, and provider and consumer interest groups often yields regulatory changes, the ultimate direction of peer review is controlled by Congress, where a handful of federal lawmakers, mostly in the House of Representatives, is concerned with the PRO program. Important players there include Pete Stark; Henry Waxman (D-Calif.), who chairs the health subcommittee of the Energy and Commerce Committee; Ralph Hall (D-Tex.), a member of the same health subcommittee; Willis D. Gradison Jr. (R-Ohio), the ranking minority member of Stark's Ways and Means health subcommittee; and Ted Weiss (D-N.Y.), the dour chairman of the House Government Operations subcommittee on human resources.

Waxman's seniority, unwavering support from voters, and key

position on the Energy and Commerce health subcommittee give him substantial clout among his colleagues. But he has sometimes disappointed PRO advocates. Despite credentials as a consumer activist that date back to tough legislation on medical malpractice that he championed in the California legislature, Waxman has tacitly sided with PRO opponent Hall. Insiders agree Hall never could have succeeded in winning special treatment for rural doctors facing PRO-backed fines or exclusions had it not been for Waxman's acquiescence. Most suspect simple horse-trading: Waxman allowed Hall's efforts to limit PRO authority in exchange for Hall's support of Waxman's 1987 nursing-home-reform legislation.

Congressmen Stark and Gradison are harder to figure. Stark can usually be counted on to favor anything the AMA opposes. A long-time critic of doctors, Stark was the target of an unprecedented 1986 attack by the AMA's political action committee. In an effort to unseat him, the PAC contributed more than $250,000 to a virtually unknown opponent. The effort failed, and Stark has since been even more antagonistic toward organized medicine. Despite his strong feelings that physicians need scrutiny, Stark has become openly skeptical of PROs' effectiveness. Both he and Gradison, his highly regarded Republican counterpart on the subcommittee, have taken to wondering out loud whether PROs have the chutzpah to make tough review decisions about local doctors. Among other things, the lawmakers have faulted PROs for poor performance on pre-procedure review. Interestingly, neither man has taken HCFA to task, as the GAO and others have, for writing the weak-kneed directives for preprocedure review that helped cause the failure.

Of the four, only Hall began as an enemy of the program. An otherwise unremarkable politician, he has tirelessly aided the Texas Medical Association in its fight with the IG and the Texas PRO over sanctions against rural physicians. Hall has sparred with Kusserow in hearing rooms and successfully sponsored budget amendments designed to protect rural practitioners. Thus, he has become an important player in PRO policy despite a minimal power base in Congress.

Many lawmakers and government officials consider Ted Weiss a trying person to deal with. While presiding over excruciatingly long hearings on what he takes to be the PROs' appalling failure to protect Medicare beneficiaries, he rarely looks up from a long list of written questions used to cross-examine witnesses. Unfortunately, Weiss has repeatedly confused records flagged for further review with confirmed problems; confused serious quality problems with documentation issues; and misinterpreted statistical analyses to make the care afforded the nation's elderly appear scandalous. Some lobbyists blame Weiss's staff for the errors.

In the Senate, interest in PROs has been less consistent. John Heinz (R-Pa.) had substantial influence that now appears to be waning. Like Kusserow, Heinz is often accused of shooting from the hip. A pet provision Heinz was able to pass in 1986 mandated PRO payment denials for substandard care. But HHS managers, not to mention consumer and provider lobbyists, pronounced the legislation unworkable as written, and it has yet to be implemented. Dave Durenberger (R-Minn.) has also been prominent in PRO politics in the past, but his influence has been weakened by charges that he evaded Senate limits on speaking fees members may receive from private groups.

This relationship between administrators, lobbies, Congress, and physicians is what makes health-care policy, and PRO policy in particular, so complicated. But congressmen and lobbyists come and go. For the physicians whose lives are affected by the day-to-day workings of the system, Morford, Kusserow, and to a lesser extent Wilensky, are the people to watch.

Given that Wilensky is a political appointee and that none of her predecessors has lasted more than four years as HCFA administrator, her influence over the PRO program may be short-lived. Kusserow, to the chagrin of his many critics and despite the efforts of the AMA, is not likely to be thrown out of office anytime soon. He has solid support from the White House, from HHS secretary Louis Sullivan, and from congressional powerhouses like Stark. But perhaps he is mellowing. Early this year AMA general counsel Kirk Johnson opined that Kusserow's *PrimeTime* fiasco last fall had moderated the IG's hostility toward organized medicine.

Morford, a career official who's wise to the ways of power in the capital, is the person most likely to have a lasting effect on the PRO system. As long as he remains in office, physicians can expect that changes in the ways PROs work will be predictable. But Morford is pushing hard for the UCDS, and his position as operations man in charge of the project could make him vulnerable. If it fails, as critics predict it will (see Chapter 8), Morford will be blamed. If it works, he'll share in the success. In the interim, physicians can expect that the PROs will continue to be run in a steady and methodical way.

CHAPTER FIVE

REVIEW CATEGORIES: HOW PROVIDERS GET TARGETED

From the beginning, day-to-day PRO activities have focused on a few key areas: review of hospital admissions for medical necessity and appropriateness; review of readmissions and transfers to detect premature discharge; review of DRG coding accuracy to find overpayments; and review of outlier cases (those with features that deviate significantly from the norm) to ascertain whether extraordinary payments were justified. The guts of the PRO review process are contained in a document known as a scope of work. HCFA has issued one scope of work for each of three federal PRO contract periods. Always a patchwork affair loaded with hard-to-understand bureaucratic lingo, the scope of work guides all PRO review activity for a given contract period.

The first scope of work (1984-86) was shaped by suspicion that certain providers would attempt to game the new Prospective Payment System by discharging patients from hospitals prematurely, transferring patients from PPS-covered beds to beds reimbursed in the traditional way, or by upcoding the diagnosis to an illness more serious—and lucrative—than the one a patient actually had. The second scope of work (1986-88) emphasized quality of care and the development of "generic quality screens," procedural checklists that PRO nurses began applying to each case they reviewed. The screens, which have since proliferated, are designed to signal potential problems with discharge planning, medical stability at discharge, unanticipated deaths, nosocomial infections, unscheduled returns to operating rooms, and inpatient trauma. Cases that fail one or more screens are usually forwarded to PRO physicians for review. During the second contract period, HCFA also required PROs to launch community-outreach efforts and mandated review of HMOs that enroll Medicare beneficiaries.

In 1988, HCFA began awarding contracts under its third scope of work, a three-year plan coinciding with the new three-year review contracts, and all PROs are now operating under its provisions (see Appendix). This scope features the Quality Intervention Plan, a sort of arithmetical demerit system for doctors. Quite simply, the QIP assigns numerical values to quality problems and requires PROs to act when health-care providers rack up a specified number of points. In addition, this round of contracts saw the beginning of pre-procedure review, ambulatory-surgery review, and review of "intervening care," which occurs when a patient is readmitted to a hospital within 31 days of the original admission.

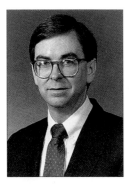

Dr. John Kelly of the AMA says the soundness of PRO review criteria varies widely from specialty to specialty.

In addition, the third scope of work requires PROs to apply quality screens to each case they review; to identify premature discharges; to ascertain that hospital admissions are necessary; to ensure that invasive procedures are "reasonable and medically necessary"; to validate DRG assignments; to review special cases in which Medicare extends coverage not normally provided; and to determine whether beneficiaries or providers should have known in advance that certain services weren't covered by Medicare.

Adverse quality findings, officially known as error rates, must be computed for each hospital on a quarterly basis. If a hospital is found to have an error rate of 5 percent or higher, with at least six cases, the PRO must begin "intensified review."

To help identify providers whose practices are consistently aberrant, PROs are expected to compile highly detailed statistical profiles of every physician and hospital that treats Medicare patients. For hospitals, PROs must keep statistics on such things as mortality rates, readmission rates, admission denial rates, rates of premature discharge, average length of stay for each DRG, and rates of generic-quality-screen failure. For physicians, PROs must maintain up-to-date statistics on denial rates for admissions and readmissions, mortality rates, and, for premature discharges, average length of stay.

Finally, PROs are required to keep statistics on internal operations. PRO physicians, nurses, and medical-records technicians must be rated on the accuracy of their review determinations and their DRG validation findings. The table on the opposite page shows the evolution of PRO review from its inception.

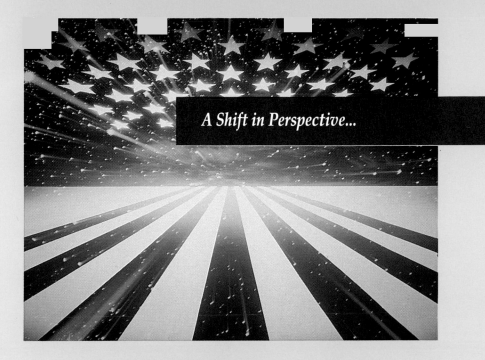

A Shift in Perspective...

Showing Our True Colors...

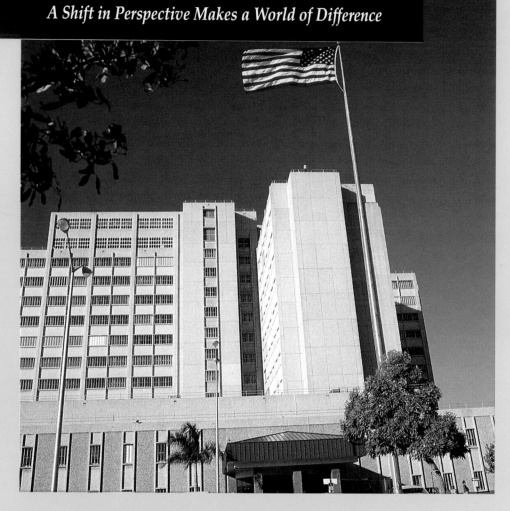

A Shift in Perspective Makes a World of Difference

Showing Our True Colors:
A Commitment to Government and Institutional Healthcare

We have a clear understanding of the needs and expectations of government and institutional healthcare providers. We recognize that value begins—but does not end—with quality products. That's why we're committed to support programs that go far beyond your expectations—continuing education programs... cooperative research...technical consultation...product information hotlines... custom packaging...and patient education. All designed to assist you in the delivery of quality healthcare. We're Marion Merrell Dow.

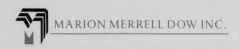

MARION MERRELL DOW INC.

Evolution of PRO Scope of Work Requirements

Must Review	1984	1986	1988
Transfers	From PPS hospital to another hospital, exempt unit, swing bed.	Same, but lower level of review.	Lower level of review of transfers from PPS to another PPS hospital, and 25 percent from PPS to exempt swing beds.
Readmissions	All related readmissions within seven days.	All related readmissions within 15 days.	25 percent of all readmissions within 31 days.
Focused DRGs	DRG 468 (unrelated operating room procedure). DRG 462 (rehabilitation) was added during the contract period.	DRG 468 (unrelated operating room procedure), DRG 462 (rehabilitation), DRG 088 (chronic obstructive pulmonary disease).	Lower level of review for DRG 462 and DRG 468. Focused review of DRG 088 is deleted. Adds 100 percent review of DRG 472 (extensive burns), DRG 474 (tracheostomy), DRG 475 (mechanical ventilation through endotracheal intubation), and seven low-volume DRGs related to newborns.
Preadmission Review	Five procedures proposed by PRO.	Pacemakers plus four procedures proposed by PRO.	100 percent review of 10 procedures (inpatient or outpatient procedures). Mandatory cataract and carotid endarterectomy surgery, plus eight other procedures proposed by PRO.
Community Outreach	Not in contracts.	All PROs to propose program.	Mandatory toll-free beneficiary hotline. Programs to inform beneficiaries about PRO review. Response to written inquiries within 30 days.
Intervening Care	Not in contracts.	Not in contracts.	Review a sample of post-hospital care (home health care, skilled nursing-facility care, hospital outpatient care) that is given between two hospital readmissions where the second admission is within 31 days of discharge of the original one.

The scope of work is enormously prescriptive, and PRO executives bridle at the rigidity and complexity of the mandatory plan. On the one hand, they're told to develop their own review objectives and focus on areas they define as worthy of close scrutiny. On the other, they're given an enormous amount of work over which they have virtually no control.

One of the more outspoken PRO executives, Edward Lynch of the Rhode Island PRO, argues that the massive work required by HCFA deprives PROs of the flexibility to focus resources on local problems. "Instead we become technocrats," he says. "For this size PRO, we have a very, very tight budget, and all of it is directed toward what we're prescribed to do in our federal contract."

There are signs that complaints like this one are getting through to HCFA leaders. In late 1990, an early draft of the fourth scope of work appeared. It proposed elimination of targeted preprocedure, readmission, and intervening-care review (i.e., mandatory review of cases within specific categories); expansion of random case selection methodology; and cuts of 10 percent to 25 percent in PRO budgets. The plan forecasts review of about 10 percent of Medicare inpatient cases, down from the historic high of 50 percent. This scope of work is not yet final.

PROs have some autonomy in developing review criteria, the written standards they use to guide nurse-reviewers in choosing cases to refer to a physician. To help nurses identify potential problems, many PROs have adopted criteria in consultation with physician specialty societies, a practice that could help organized medicine and the PROs avoid many future conflicts. The AMA's Dr. Kelly for example, praises the wide use of "very solid" screening criteria for cardiac pacemakers developed by the American College of Cardiology. But he also notes instances in which criteria have been developed with little or no information from specialty groups. One example, he says, involved a PRO that developed anesthesiology guidelines on the basis of a single physician's judgment. "If anesthesiologists had followed certain portions of those criteria," Dr. Kelly says, "patients would have been injured. Fortunately, the shortcomings of those criteria were identified fairly rapidly and necessary changes were made."

The current HCFA workplan directs PROs to circulate criteria to state medical societies for comment and to provide them to anyone who asks. This is in contrast to the practice of utilization-review companies that work for insurers and corporations. Such firms typically limit release of criteria to physicians appealing specific cases.

Under the third scope of work, the logistics of how PROs draw their review samples are fairly complicated. First, insurance companies that process Medicare Part A claims regularly send computerized billing information to each PRO. The PRO examines these data tapes and selects cases—sometimes randomly, sometimes using predetermined review categories. Once cases are chosen, nurse-reviewers request photocopies of the medical records or view them at the hospital. The nurses use the written review criteria to screen each record, and when a case is considered questionable, it goes to a physician-reviewer, who must be a licensed doctor with an active practice and admitting privileges at one or more hospitals in the PRO service area.

If the physician-reviewer determines that all or part of a payment shouldn't be made, the attending physician receives an "initial denial notice" and has the opportunity to respond within 20 days. Failure to respond or failure to persuade the PRO physician to change his or her determination results in a "payment denial notice," which is sent to the beneficiary, physician or other provider, and fiscal intermediary. The intermediary then adjusts the hospital payment.

If the denied payment is for unnecessary surgery, the surgeon's fee is denied as well. This requires communication between the Part A and Part B intermediaries. If the denial involves a medical admission, the Part B carrier is notified, but it may exercise some discretion on whether to deny payment to the treating physician— a doctor may be paid even when the hospital isn't, on the grounds that although the patient required treatment, it need not have been provided in an acute-care setting.

A beneficiary, physician, or other provider may request PRO reconsideration of a payment denial within 60 days of the first denial notice. If possible, reconsiderations must be decided by PRO physician-reviewers, preferably board-certified in the same specialty as the treating physician. The reconsideration cannot be decided by the physician who reviewed the case initially. Beneficiaries who are awaiting admission or who are inpatients may file requests for expedited reconsiderations within three days of a denial notice. Because PROs overturn payment-denial decisions more than 40 percent of the time, wise physicians almost always file for a PRO reconsideration. Hospitals have also learned this lesson. PROs say some now routinely appeal every denial.

It's possible to appeal an unfavorable reconsideration, but the process is difficult. In most cases, only beneficiaries may originate such an appeal, and it must involve a payment of more than $200. These appeals are heard by administrative law judges employed by the Social Security Administration. If the amount contested is at least $2,000, then an adverse decision by an administrative law judge can be appealed further to a three-member appeals council. Doctors and hospitals contend that these rules are unfair because, in most instances, beneficiaries, who suffer no financial loss if payment is denied, are the only parties who can appeal adverse reconsideration decisions. Why, they ask, can't appeals be filed by the parties directly affected? So far, such arguments haven't persuaded Congress to change the law.

Denial rates (not including reconsiderations) vary widely. The average hospital payment-denial rate for all PROs for the 35-month period that ended in May 1989 was 2.31 percent. PROs with higher-than-average rates included the Virgin Islands (7.95 percent); the District of Columbia (5.14 percent); South Carolina (4.9 percent); and Illinois (4.76 percent). PROs with the lowest denial rates were Oklahoma (0.63 percent); Hawaii (1.18 percent); and North Carolina (1.29 percent).

More recent statistics, which offer comparisons among review categories, suggest that denial rates are declining. The average inpatient hospital denial rate for reviews completed from April 1 through December 31, 1989, was 2.01 percent. Among PROs with caseloads of 6,000 or more, the District of Columbia PRO continued to have a relatively high denial rate (5.13 percent), followed by PROs in Connecticut (4.02 percent) and Utah (3.79 percent). The national preprocedure denial rate was only 0.17 percent. Ambulatory-surgery denials were 0.70 percent, and the vast majority of those came from one review group, the Massachusetts PRO. A child of the Massachusetts Medical Society, that PRO says its rates are high not because it's overly aggressive, but because it was one of the first to use review criteria from the third scope of work and was given different instructions on how to calculate denials (the Massachusetts PRO is now reporting much lower denial rates).

Despite apprehensions to the contrary, the most important thing to remember about PRO payment denial rates is that they started out low and are declining. HCFA's published findings through the end of June 1990 show hospital denials dipping below 2 percent, to a nationwide average of 1.92 percent. The same holds true for preprocedure review: denials fell from a tiny rate of 0.17 percent to an even tinier 0.15 percent. Ambulatory-surgery denial rates slipped from 0.70 percent to 0.59 percent. Finally, for inpatient denials, there's the issue of reversals following appeals. HCFA isn't anxious to advertise this, and it has yet to integrate these findings into final denial tabulations, but as noted, PROs reverse hospital payment denials in four of every 10 appealed cases. And about a third of all inpatient denials are appealed.

Adverse quality determinations are a different matter. Though these don't yet carry direct financial penalties, they do result in black marks against physicians and can trigger substantial PRO interventions. Although the rates for adverse quality determinations appear to be falling as well—inpatient findings were down to a nationwide average of 1.83 percent through June 1990—the effects of such findings can be quite damaging, even catastrophic, to a physician's practice.

CHAPTER SIX

QUALITY INTERVENTIONS: RATING DOCTORS

T he Quality Intervention Plan mandated by the third scope of work is even more controversial than PROs' payment denial authority. The QIP was designed to ensure that all PROs actually intervene when they detect care of dubious quality (HCFA strongly suspected some weren't doing so). The new initiative created a point system that automatically mandates actions at predetermined levels.

Before a physician accrues points for poor quality of care, however, a long chain of events must occur. The process begins with the generic quality screens that PRO nurses use to detect deviations from professionally recognized standards. Screens for hospital care are designed to flag problems with discharge planning, medical stability at discharge, unexpected deaths, nosocomial infections, unscheduled returns to surgery, and trauma. Generic quality screens for home health agency care monitor adequacy of intake evaluation, appropriate and timely interventions, adequacy of restorative care, deaths within 48 hours of transfer to a hospital, secondary infections, complications, documentation of plans for follow-up care, and provision of a discharge summary to the physician of record. In addition to these generic quality screens, PROs use uniform quality checklists to evaluate care provided in hospital outpatient departments, skilled nursing facilities, ambulatory-surgery centers, and psychiatric programs.

When a screen yields a discrepancy in care, the nurse-reviewer refers the case to a physician-adviser. The adviser reviews the case using his or her own best clinical judgment, regardless of screen findings. If the physician sees a potential quality problem, the case usually goes for review to a specialist in the appropriate field, or to a committee that includes such a specialist.

If the findings of the second review agree with the first, the health-care provider is notified. Failure to respond, or failure to persuade the PRO that it has erred, results in a "confirmed quality problem," designated as level one, two, or three. Level one problems, which count for one point on a physician's record, are those without potential to harm a patient; level two problems (five points) are those found to have potential adverse effects; level three problems (25 points) involve "significant adverse effects on the patient."

Physicians who receive at least one but fewer than nine points in a given quarter are notified of their infractions only to help them avoid future points. For totals between 10 and 14 points, the PRO must require specific educational efforts, such as a review of the literature, continuing medical education, or self-education. Totals of 15 points or more require the PRO to review every Medicare hospital case the physician has treated in the time period or, if an institution is held responsible, every case in the appropriate category. Totals exceeding 20 points demand additional action, such as mandatory preadmission review, referral to a hospital committee, or monitoring of a physician's cases by a colleague on staff at a hospital. And when a provider's quality demerits exceed 25 in a given quarter, the PRO must consider a sanction recommendation and notification of licensing authorities.

In general, points are computed on a quarterly basis. The history of all infractions is maintained from quarter to quarter. PROs are no longer required to discuss and make final decisions on every level one finding. Instead, the PRO may allow level one points to stand until a pattern emerges. Three level one screen failures in one quarter trigger a discussion with the physician, as do five level one points in two quarters.

And, while penalties for level one infractions usually last no more than one quarter, those for levels two and three may require that the physician be put on a continuing corrective-action plan that lasts more than one quarter. Thus, evaluations made during one quarter may, at the PRO's discretion, result in PRO monitoring for longer than one quarter.

So far, the QIP hasn't created an avalanche of actions against physicians. As noted earlier, of about 1.5 million reviews completed by December 31, 1989, 2.3 percent were found to have confirmed quality problems. And among confirmed problems, the vast majority were level one (documentation) infractions.

Nonetheless, physicians are understandably anxious about their performance ratings—anxious enough that, in some cases, they react to a notice of points in a manner that may be self-defeating. The AMA recommends that doctors who receive a citation of potential quality problems follow a five-step process. Borrowing a page from manuals on earthquakes and nuclear attacks, the group first advises doctors to "keep calm. Do not send angry letters to the PRO; discuss the quality issue with a peer." Second, the AMA prescribes a careful review of the medical record at issue to determine whether the PRO has made a simple factual error or missed a favorable piece of documentation. The group warns against telephoning the PRO. It urges doctors to communicate in writing "without self-serving statements, argumentative remarks, explicit or implicit admissions of error in judgment, or criticism of care provided by others." The AMA notes that physicians have the right to request personal interviews with PRO physicians and, in complex cases, suggests doing this before writing. Finally, the group recommends that all PRO correspondence be kept in a file separate from the medical record. This is to assure confidentiality in the event that the record is subpoenaed.

One stumbling block for QIP has been assigning points when blame is hard to place. This is especially tricky in academic settings, where potential culprits may include the physician, the hospital, the resident, and the academic program that trained the resident. The issue has been especially hot in New York, where hospital and physician groups have opposed QIP on the grounds that it assigns point scores and disciplinary actions against physicians in training, who, by definition, are expected to make mistakes.

Teaching hospitals argue that they risk being held responsible for adverse determinations against medical residents who may ignore a PRO letter or who have been moved to a different clinical rotation and never receive it. Teaching physicians worry that if the resident isn't blamed, then the attending physician will be. Pro bono attendings have vocally denounced a system in which they may be racking up PRO points for cases handled by their residents.

By the end of 1990, HCFA still hadn't devised a solution, though it had considered several options. One of the most popular was discussed during a huddle between physician and hospital representatives held at HCFA's Baltimore headquarters in September 1990.

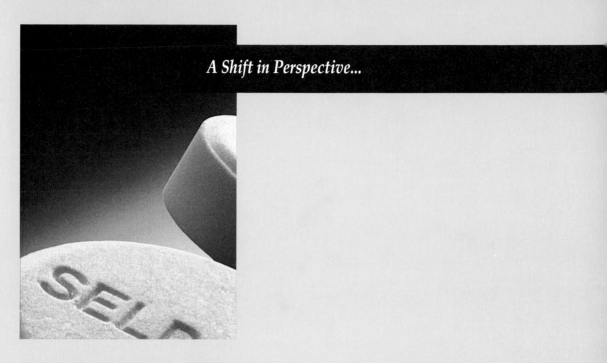

Behind Every Seldane Tablet...

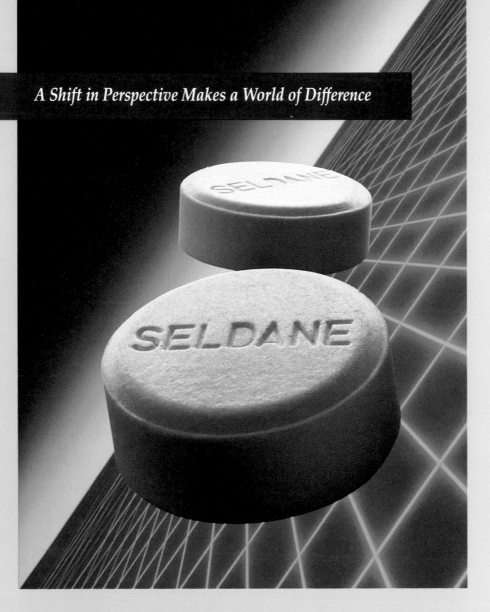

A Shift in Perspective Makes a World of Difference

A Commitment to Allergy

Beyond the welcome revolution in allergy treatment, SELDANE has given Marion Merrell Dow the opportunity to provide extraordinary support and services to the field of Allergy. Financial support of education. Sponsorship of meetings. Scholarship awards. Symposia and lecture series. And the ongoing, innovative research that is shifting perspectives in the treatment of a wide range of allergy-related conditions.

From any perspective, SELDANE adds breadth and depth to the world of the Allergist.

SELDANE®
(terfenadine) 60 mg tablets

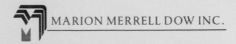

MARION MERRELL DOW INC.

Representatives of academic medicine suggested that problems with physicians in training should trigger a corrective action plan designed by the teaching program. Hospital quality-assurance departments would make sure residents received PRO determinations and responded to them. Pro bono attendings would be held responsible only when they provided direct patient care.

But technical dilemmas like this may prove the least of HCFA's worries over QIP. One of the ablest critics of the PRO program, Philadelphia provider attorney Alice Gosfield, argues that the Quality Intervention Plan is inherently unfair, an "internally self-validating mechanism" that offers little recourse to its targets. Unlike PRO sanctions, for which there are numerous appeal mechanisms, the QIP offers no opportunity for external oversight, she says. A practitioner can be required to undergo what Gosfield calls "de facto sanctions"—self-education, formal continuing medical education, or even a mini-residency program—without being given the opportunity to appeal. The PRO has all the power in such a system because failure to submit to corrective action can be viewed as grounds for considering a sanction and because, says Gosfield, "frequently the punishment doesn't fit the crime."

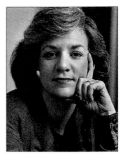

Alice Gosfield is a Philadelphia health-care attorney and a critic of the PRO system.

Predictably, HCFA's Morford disagrees—strongly. No fan of attorneys—they would like to strangle the entire process with red tape, he alleges—the government's PRO chief argues that the QIP is merely a method for bringing substandard physicians up to par and returning them to the practice of mainstream medicine, the very essence of local peer review. "We're trying to get doctors to talk to one another," he says.

HCFA also argues that it needed some way to galvanize PROs that are reluctant to take tough corrective action against doctors who are known to have problems. A case in point involved the former contract holder for the New York PRO, accused of repeatedly failing to act on its own findings of substandard quality (see Chapter 2). Forced into competitive bidding, the PRO lost its contract to one of its own subcontractors in December 1989. PRO program managers hope the numerical approach will bring substandard review groups into line without the need to rebid contracts.

But no action will be of value if PROs aren't detecting infractions. "I personally feel quality problems are higher than what the PROs are finding," says Richard Husk, HSQB's director of medical review. This view is bolstered by statistics from the superPRO, the organization that rereviews the reports of local PROs.

In late 1990, statistics were published that compared superPRO findings with those of 13 PROs. The comparison showed that the superPRO questioned quality in roughly 10 percent of 2,706 inpatient cases to which PROs had given passing grades. That result wasn't necessarily unexpected, given that the superPRO doesn't interact with local physicians and thus doesn't hear treating physicians' explanations. What *was* unexpected was that PROs did not contest the superPRO's decisions in fully 48 percent of cases in which findings differed. The PROs essentially conceded they'd missed about half of the problems they should have detected.

That finding prompted Morford to deliver an angry lecture on contract responsibilities to PRO representatives attending an AMPRA meeting in Chicago. "I'm not interested in targets, but I am interested in [PROs' making] the right decisions," he told the group.

If PRO review of hospital care has been a headache for program officials, the attempt to monitor care in health maintenance organizations qualifies as a migraine. Congress extended PROs' authority to review HMO records in 1987 over the strenuous opposition of the prepaid-health-care industry. More and more Medicare beneficiaries were choosing to become members of HMOs, and lawmakers feared that the HMOs' vaunted cost-control strategies would result in undertreatment of frail elderly patients. Those fears were intensified by a scandal that involved gross mismanagement at the enormous International Medical Centers in Florida, which enrolled tens of thousands of elderly patients before being bought by Humana Inc. in 1987. HMOs were wary too. Many had declined to get into the Medicare business, and those that had signed up were quick to suggest that PRO physician-advisers had a fee-for-service mentality that prevented them from understanding how alternative delivery systems operate. Some also worried that PRO physicians would vent their own competitive biases to create distrust among the public.

After a number of legislative thrusts and parries, Congress authorized PRO review of a sample of records representing the roughly one million Medicare patients enrolled in HMOs nationally. HCFA reluctantly drew up a review scheme. Factions within the agency worried that PROs lacked the expertise to perform this sort of review competently, and that aggressive review might further discourage HMOs from enrolling Medicare patients, derailing a program that both the Reagan and Bush administrations had strongly advocated.

The HCFA plan's emphasis was on detecting undertreatment;

PROs were told to focus on hospitalizations of HMO Medicare patients. Immediately, arcane logistical problems developed, and PROs had difficulty obtaining HMO inpatient medical records. Some analysts blame hospital foot-dragging; some blame HMOs; some point to the insurance companies that process hospital bills. Whatever the reason, the result has been fewer HMO inpatient reviews than anticipated.

Attempts to gather ambulatory patient records from independ-ent-practice HMOs were even more frustrating. These loose con-federations of physicians practicing in private offices are the type of HMO most often accused of lacking effective quality-assurance programs. Because the groups often have no central record-keeping system, ambulatory patient records must be obtained from the physician's private office. Not surprisingly, the process is time-con-suming and costly, and doctors see it as an intrusion.

HCFA hadn't publicly distributed any HMO review statistics as of early 1991, so it's not known whether PROs are uncovering a substantial percentage of quality problems there (although a leaked document prepared in 1989 showed such problems in the 4 per-cent range). Cynics blame the lack of information on politics, claiming that HCFA is refusing to release statistics to protect the HMO industry. HCFA is more interested in increasing Medicare HMO enrollment, they argue, than in demonstrating PRO oversight. Others say the explanation is less sinister: they allege that HCFA botched its PRO data-reporting system for HMO review and doesn't really have much to report. Rather than open itself to embarrassing questions about its own performance, runs this argument, the agency has simply decided to stonewall.

Comments from some federal officials confirm that HMO review has not gone as planned. "We don't know how valid anything we now see is," concedes HSQB's Husk. "We've had one and a half years of trouble with the system. I'll be honest about that."

Anecdotal evidence suggests that PRO review of HMOs hasn't uncovered any smoking guns. Husk claims adverse quality findings against HMOs are running in the 3 percent range—only slightly higher than the rate for fee-for-service medicine. Moreover, a high-er rate is to be expected because HMO review is more extensive and tracks patients beyond single encounters. Statistics released by the California PROs show HMO quality problems in the 1 percent range, hardly a cause for alarm. Perhaps most telling, no sanctions have been imposed against an HMO by the IG's office following a PRO investigation.

As of early 1991, PROs weren't yet routinely denying payment when they found evidence of substandard quality. Under the original PRO law, review groups had the authority to deny payment only for services judged inappropriate or unnecessary (utilization review). In a federal budget bill passed in 1986, Congress tried to add the authority to routinely deny payments for substandard care (quality review). The law, which was supposed to take effect immediately, proved extraordinarily controversial. As a result, HCFA didn't even publish a "proposed rule" until January 1989.

The controversy centered on the patient-notification portion of the 1986 law. The section said that when PROs detected poor-quality care, and before the physician had been offered the right to a rereview, they were to notify the patient as well as the physician or provider. The notification was to take the form of a letter to the patient stating that "the quality of services you received does not meet professionally recognized standards of health care."

It didn't take long for experts to recognize the malpractice implications of such letters. One Washington lobbyist referred to that provision as a bill of rights for the malpractice bar. Obviously, any such direct communication from a federally directed review entity to a patient would constitute powerful grounds for a lawsuit. Attorneys wouldn't have to hunt for experts to criticize a physician's performance; they'd have the critique in writing, courtesy of the local PRO!

The AMA strenuously opposed implementing the law, despite assurances from the AARP that retirees rarely sue. In the end, HCFA was apprehensive enough to quietly shelve its regulations. Even the law's sponsor, Senator Heinz, acquiesced in the do-nothing strategy. A partial solution was reached when a House-Senate conference committee included a fix in the 1989 federal budget bill. The letter to the patient would be sent only after the physician had been offered the right to a rereview of the case by a specialist. Assuming the second review confirmed the deficiency, the text of the beneficiary letter would be watered down to state only that "the medical care received was not acceptable under the Medicare program." No longer would it include a reference to care not meeting recognized standards.

On the books since 1986, the subject of a proposed rule in January 1989, and revised in December 1989, PROs' authority to deny payment for substandard quality was scheduled to be implemented in 1991. One legal scholar who has studied the program calls HCFA's delay in implementing the law "unconscionable" and perhaps illegal. But no one has taken the government to court.

Whereas payment denials, quality interventions, and denials for substandard quality all have (or will have) significant implications for physicians treating Medicare patients, they pale in comparison with the PROs' sanction authority. As discussed earlier, sanctions can result in a physician's being suspended from the Medicare program indefinitely or for a fixed number of years. Lesser problems can result in fines. In either case, a physician or provider risks having his or her name published in a local newspaper, along with a description of the finding. All parties agree that public notices can have catastrophic consequences for a medical practice.

Sanctions, which have been around since shortly after the inception of the PRO program in the early 1980s, continue to be the subject of wide misunderstanding. PROs themselves have no authority to fine or suspend a physician, hospital, ambulatory-surgery center, HMO, home health agency, or skilled nursing facility. That authority rests solely with the inspector general. What PROs can do is *recommend* actions against providers. It's up to the IG's office to act. And, despite the perception of many physicians, the IG frequently refuses to accept PRO recommendations (usually on procedural grounds) or reduces the severity of a proposed punishment. But the IG can impose a more severe penalty than the PRO has recommended, although this has never happened.

Under federal law, PROs can recommend fines or suspensions against physicians or other providers for one or more instances of having "grossly and flagrantly" violated professional obligations to Medicare patients. They can also recommend sanctions if a practitioner "failed in a substantial number of cases substantially to comply" with quality standards. A PRO considering a sanction on either ground must inform the provider in writing, via a "potential sanction notice." This is followed by an informal meeting between the PRO and the provider. The accused provider may bring an attorney to the meeting, but it isn't a formal legal proceeding, and the attorney isn't permitted to cross-examine a PRO physician. The outcome of a meeting may be that the PRO and the physician agree on a corrective plan, though the PRO isn't required to offer one.

A PRO that has met with the provider or physician and intends to ask for a sanction must submit its recommendation and all pertinent evidence in writing to the inspector general. The IG then has 120 days to act. Failure to act results in automatic imposition of the PRO recommendation until the IG does act. The IG's office prides itself, though, on never having failed to act within the time period. Sanctions may be, and often are, appealed to HHS administrative law judges. Beyond that, they can be brought up before an appeals council of three administrative law judges and, if a target wishes, can be appealed again in federal court (see charts on pages 47 and 49).

Sanctions hinge on the critical issue of a provider's "unwillingness or lack of ability" to improve in the future. Regardless of the severity of the problems, the IG's office isn't supposed to take action unless it's convinced that a physician or provider is either unwilling or unable to comply with professionally recognized standards. To a large extent then, the IG is put into the position of trying to read the practitioner's state of mind.

Patton and others—notably the consumer advocate Dr. Sidney Wolfe and the AARP—have urged the deletion of the "unwillingness or lack of ability" clause from the PRO law on the grounds that a physician's actions are at issue, not whether he or she promises to do better in the future. So far they've been unsuccessful. Groups such as the AMA and the Texas Medical Association have successfully argued that sanctions should be considered only as a last resort and ought not to be imposed if there's a chance the practitioner can be reeducated. In 1990 Congress passed legislation directing PROs to order corrective action plans, if possible, before recommending sanctions against a physician. This was done as a way to clarify whether the physician seemed willing or able to improve.

In part because of the need to show that a provider is unwilling or unable to improve, a physician's chances of being kicked out of Medicare are remote. From 1985 through August 1990, PROs submitted 224 sanction recommendations to the IG's office. They resulted in the exclusion from Medicare of 95 doctors and one hospital; 25 physicians and two hospitals were fined. The IG rejected 87 cases: 33 because of procedural lapses; 14 because of faulty medical evidence; and 38 because the PRO failed to prove the provider was beyond reform. The two remaining cases were closed because the physicians died before the IG could act.

Since a targeted physician's state of mind is critical in determining whether he or she ought to be sanctioned, provider attorneys agree on the tactical importance for physicians of meeting with a PRO and showing contrition, if it is merited. Doctors who ignore PRO letters or refuse to meet with review physicians are probably

PRO/HHS Sanction Process for Substantial Violations*

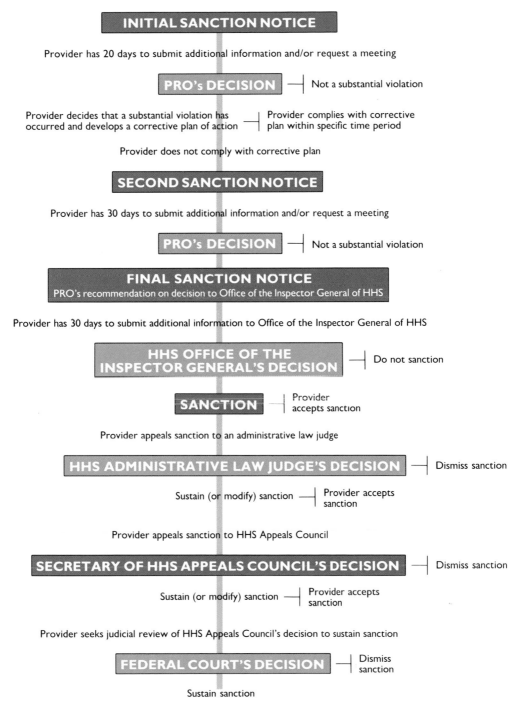

INITIAL SANCTION NOTICE

Provider has 20 days to submit additional information and/or request a meeting

PRO's DECISION — Not a substantial violation

Provider decides that a substantial violation has occurred and develops a corrective plan of action — Provider complies with corrective plan within specific time period

Provider does not comply with corrective plan

SECOND SANCTION NOTICE

Provider has 30 days to submit additional information and/or request a meeting

PRO's DECISION — Not a substantial violation

FINAL SANCTION NOTICE
PRO's recommendation on decision to Office of the Inspector General of HHS

Provider has 30 days to submit additional information to Office of the Inspector General of HHS

HHS OFFICE OF THE INSPECTOR GENERAL'S DECISION — Do not sanction

SANCTION — Provider accepts sanction

Provider appeals sanction to an administrative law judge

HHS ADMINISTRATIVE LAW JUDGE'S DECISION — Dismiss sanction

Sustain (or modify) sanction — Provider accepts sanction

Provider appeals sanction to HHS Appeals Council

SECRETARY OF HHS APPEALS COUNCIL'S DECISION — Dismiss sanction

Sustain (or modify) sanction — Provider accepts sanction

Provider seeks judicial review of HHS Appeals Council's decision to sustain sanction

FEDERAL COURT'S DECISION — Dismiss sanction

Sustain sanction

*A substantial violation is a pattern of care over a substantial number of cases that is inappropriate, unnecessary, does not meet recognized patterns of care, or is not supported by the documentation of care required by the PRO.

SOURCE: Adapted with permission from the Office of Technology Assessment, 1988

damaging their cases, perhaps irreparably.

A look at past sanction cases shows how important the doctor's actions during the sanction process can be. Take, for instance, the case of a Midwestern practitioner excluded from Medicare for five years upon the recommendation of the local PRO. In upholding the sanction in a decision published in January 1990, an administrative law judge cited "gross and flagrant abuse" of four patients, including failure to order timely blood cultures for a patient with septicemia, failure to restrict intravenous fluids in a patient with congestive heart failure, and ordering an inappropriate combination of anti-arrhythmic medications without testing blood levels for those medications. Faced with these findings in a 1988 meeting with the PRO, the physician was quoted as stating, "As long as I am practicing in Iowa I'm going to do things the way I think is best." Such a statement indicated "contempt for the peer-review system," according to the judge, and showed the physician's unwillingness to change.

Because a physician's professional reputation is at stake, it's not surprising sanctions are the most contentious and politicized element of the PRO program. Groups like the California Medical Association have accused the IG of having a "scalp in the belt" mentality when it comes to disciplining doctors. Kusserow, in turn, has criticized PROs for bringing what he claims are too few cases to act on. At the same time, PROs and the IG have been attacked for what AMA executive vice-president James Todd used to call "doctor bashing."

In the mid-1980s, battle lines were drawn over the relatively high level of sanction activity by the Texas PRO against physicians in isolated rural areas. The Texas Medical Association led the fight against the PRO, arguing that these actions were effectively depriving small communities of access to necessary medical care. The TMA lobbied Representative Hall, who succeeded in inserting language into a 1987 federal budget bill that would permit rural physicians to exercise their rights of appeal before, rather than after, the imposition of a sanction. Under the Hall provision (which became law), physicians in counties of fewer than 70,000 residents may continue to treat Medicare patients while awaiting an administrative law judge's ruling on the merits of a sanction.

Groups such as the PROs, AMPRA, and the AARP contend the Hall provision imposes a double standard that's ultimately dangerous for patients residing in those rural areas. But so far, these groups have been unsuccessful in overturning the law.

A certain equilibrium may have been achieved in the struggle between PRO advocates and opponents. The forces opposing re-

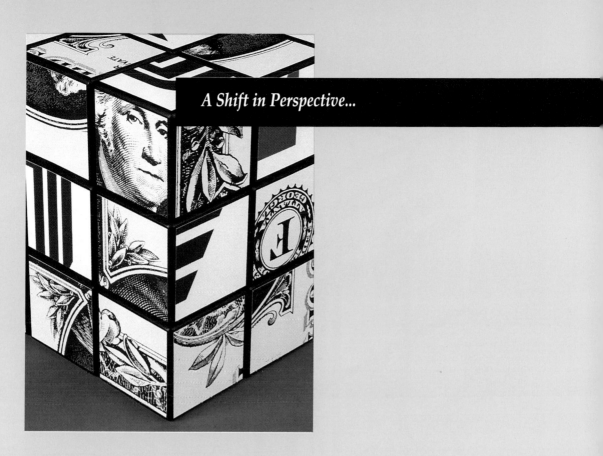

Do It Right the First Time...

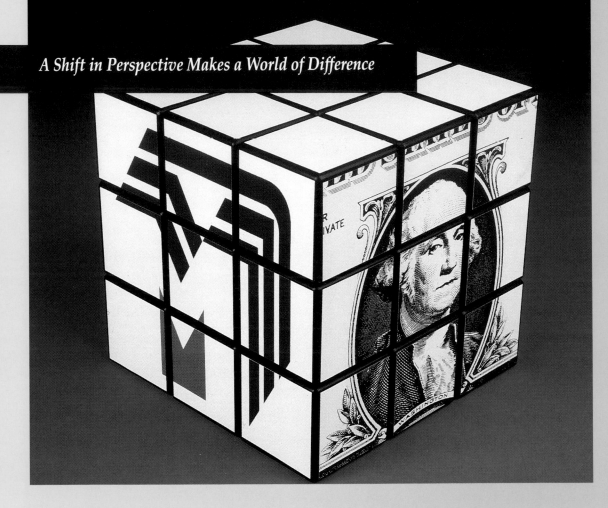

When You Do It Right the First Time...
That's Savings!

Bargains can be deceiving, appearing to achieve savings when they're
actually costing you extra time and money. We offer pharmaceuticals with
distinct, direct benefits to your patients and your facility. Unsurpassed efficacy.
Favorable side effect profiles. These translate into lower total patient costs.
Add to that our uncommon level of involvement—business-based programs,
professional programs, patient education programs. We think you'll agree that
that's uncommon commitment...uncommon value.

PRO/HHS Sanction Process for Gross and Flagrant Violations*

INITIAL SANCTION NOTICE

Provider has 30 days to submit additional information and/or request a meeting

PRO's DECISION — Not a gross and flagrant violation

FINAL SANCTION NOTICE
PRO's recommendation on decision to Office of the Inspector General of HHS

Provider has 30 days to submit additional information to the Office of the Inspector General

HHS OFFICE OF THE INSPECTOR GENERAL'S DECISION — Do not sanction

SANCTION — Provider accepts sanction

Provider appeals sanction to an administrative law judge of HHS

ADMINISTRATIVE LAW JUDGE'S DECISION — Dismiss sanction

Sustain (or modify) — Provider accepts sanction

Provider appeals sanction to HHS Appeals Council

SECRETARY OF HHS APPEALS COUNCIL'S DECISION — Dismiss sanction

Sustain (or modify) — Provider accepts sanction

Provider seeks judicial review of HHS Appeals Council's decision to sustain sanction

FEDERAL COURT'S DECISION — Dismiss sanction

Sustain sanction

*A gross and flagrant violation is a violation that has occurred in one or more instances and presents an imminent danger to the health, safety, or well-being of a Medicare beneficiary.

SOURCE: Adapted with permission from the Office of Technology Assessment, 1988

view aren't likely to abolish sanctions, while those who want tougher provisions aren't likely to weaken protections for physicians who demonstrate they're willing and able to change.

In addition, sanctions no longer generate the heat they did in the mid- to late 1980s. Why? One reason is fairly simple: the rate at which PROs recommend such actions has fallen dramatically. In the 10 months previous to September 1, 1990, PROs recommended sanctions in just 13 cases, and the IG turned down six of them. Some observers argue that PROs no longer have the stomach for protracted battles with local physicians and have been subtly pressured by HCFA (and not so subtly by the AMA) to educate rather than punish. Others point to costly and time-consuming procedural hurdles. Because of a technicality in the law, a fine can never be more than the cost of the disputed service, which may be as little as $67. That's hardly an incentive for a PRO to go through the headaches of an investigative process that can take as long as two years.

Whatever the reason, a U.S. physician has never faced more than a slim chance of being sanctioned by the feds, even for care that is clearly substandard. And the chance is even slimmer now that it was in the mid-1980s. Nonetheless, physicians know that the PROs are watching them. The question is, who's watching the PROs?

CHAPTER SEVEN

ALLEGATIONS OF PRO FRAUD

Are PROs honest? For the vast majority, the answer would seem to be yes. No fraud charges have ever been brought against 52 of the nation's 54 PROs. But in the late 1980s, to the consternation of supporters and the delight of enemies, two PROs faced federal inquiries that have had serious repercussions for the entire program. The California PRO, the nation's largest, and the Florida PRO, ranked in the top five, have been accused in federal court of faking Medicare reviews they were contractually obligated to perform.

The cases have embarrassed federal program managers in Baltimore and in the San Francisco and Atlanta regional offices. The headlines generated have diverted attention from the program's goals and heightened suspicions among many doctors and hospitals that PROs are not to be trusted. Worse, the allegations of misdoing originated not with disgruntled physicians or providers holding a grudge against review groups, but with whistle-blowers—employees of the PROs themselves—who said they wished only to expose the truth. Of course, those employees (two in California and two in Florida) also stand to gain a substantial portion of whatever the government collects if the cases are proved or settled out of court. The federal False Claims Act, first passed during the Civil War, was amended in 1986 to offer protection and incentives to employees who provide information that might not otherwise reach prosecutors. Under its terms, whistle-blowers who offer information judged critical to a subsequent civil action stand to receive between 15 percent and 25 percent of whatever the government collects in damages. Lawmakers passed this amendment amid concern over questionable billing practices by Department of Defense contractors, and it's fair to assume they didn't expect to see it used against watchdog groups like PROs, which are themselves charged with monitoring questionable billing practices by health-care providers.

The California case began in the fall of 1987, when a middle-level PRO employee and former career Army officer told the U.S. Attorney's office in San Francisco that the California PRO had been paid thousands of dollars for cases it had never reviewed. The whistleblower alleged that the PRO, under pressure to complete a backlog of work, secretly dumped cases and then pretended it had reviewed them. Another employee claimed to have seen thousands of review summaries, indicating that all the reviews had been completed over a couple of days, logged on to the PRO's computer system. The employees claimed the PRO couldn't possibly have done the reviews in such a short period.

The U.S. Attorney referred the case to the regional office of the HHS inspector general to investigate. Ironically, the same office had already processed numerous sanction recommendations by the California PRO, at one time the nation's most aggressive. Meanwhile, Justice joined the whistle-blowers in false-claims and breach-of-contract actions that were unsealed in federal court in March 1989. The suit charged the PRO with billing HCFA for 51,094 reviews that were never completed. The suit also alleged that the PRO submitted four payment invoices to HCFA "knowing them to contain false or fraudulent representations . . . or acting with reckless disregard or deliberate ignorance thereof." Named in the complaint were four senior PRO officials, including the chief executive officer.

Speaking through its attorneys, the PRO at first denounced the government's case and strongly denied the allegations. It later softened a bit, claiming that if too few reviews had been done in some months, too many had been done in others; and that, in any event, HCFA had specifically approved the behavior that the Justice Department was now questioning. Meanwhile, Justice launched a criminal investigation into the conduct of at least one senior employee of the California PRO.

That investigation led to charges in June 1989 that a single employee identification number—a number belonging to senior vice-president and former review director Alan Snodgrass—appeared on 30,000 of the more than 50,000 computerized review summaries at issue. A criminal grand jury indicted Snodgrass in January 1990. He pleaded innocent to the charges, but by early 1991 he was still facing two counts of making false statements—felonies that together carry a prison term of up to 10 years in jail and a fine of up to $500,000.

The PRO defended Snodgrass at the time of his indictment and allowed him to take a paid leave of absence. When he formally resigned his position in the summer of 1990, the PRO had no comment. In September 1990, Dr. Kenneth Mills, a former PRO board member, revealed that Snodgrass had been given a lump-sum payment in addition to the customary severance pay. Dr. Mills, a San Francisco internist, said the board had authorized a payment of $200,000. The PRO countered that the actual payment was less than that, and that it was meant only to cover the costs of Snodgrass' legal defense. But the group admitted that its former employee would be allowed to keep the money if he pleaded guilty. Dr. Mills argued that the open-ended nature of the payment created at least the appearance of an inducement for the employee to plead guilty, thereby saving the PRO the money and embarrassment that a trial would have entailed. Defending the payment as ethical, the PRO said Justice had pushed it to get rid of Snodgrass in order to settle the civil case against the PRO itself—pressure that is questionable in its own right, if true.

By fall, a settlement was in the works for the civil case against the PRO. A proposed out-of-court settlement—signed by the PRO, Justice, and HHS on September 13, 1990—required the PRO to pay the government $1.2 million though admitting no liability. The PRO also agreed to submit to an HCFA "contract integrity compliance program."

Word of the proposed out-of-court settlement sent the California whistle-blowers into a tizzy. One called it a "sweetheart deal" between HCFA and the PRO, intended to limit damages and avoid further embarrassment for either party. The whistle-blowers' attorney, Stuart Buckley, noted that Justice had originally estimated it would collect $6.7 million in damages. That figure might have been trebled by a successful prosecution, and Buckley claimed the government—and his clients—might ultimately have been eligible to share in more than $20 million, instead of the $1.2 million provided by the proposed settlement. The whistle-blowers want to know how the government made its loss calculations. There's no formula for estimating what the alleged fraud cost the government, and because Justice doesn't have the expertise to make such calculations, it called on HCFA for help. Thus, the victim of the alleged fraud is helping to develop estimates of its own loss. Critics say HCFA low-balled the estimate to save itself additional embarrassment. HCFA denies this.

The settlement is still subject to approval by a San Francisco federal judge, and the whistle-blowers are urging the court to reject it. They maintain the deal fails to include punishment for the PRO's failure to monitor quality of care in the 51,094 disputed cases, and they want the government to punish the four executives named in the civil suit. The whistle-blowers' critics suggest their only motive is a bigger payoff. Privately, the California PRO and some HCFA officials continue to claim that the PRO is the victim of a vendetta by employees and HHS gumshoes with vivid imaginations. Publicly, on the advice of counsel, the PRO keeps its mouth shut.

On the face of it, the civil case against the Florida PRO appears less damaging. In this case, also launched by two employee whistle-blowers, the PRO is accused of having reversed 212 initial payment-denial decisions without first conducting rereviews. The PRO had a backlog of unreviewed appeals that so irritated the Florida Hospital Association that it helped 100 member hospitals originate a suit demanding action. In charges unsealed in August 1989, the Justice Department charged that the PRO faked the rereviews to comply with an out-of-court settlement of that suit, which had required the PRO to clean up the backlog. Justice also accused the Florida PRO of backdating the faked rereviews to indicate they'd been completed within the time prescribed by the settlement agreement. The PRO denied the latter charge; its attorney called the backdating allegation "scandalous and impertinent."

More bad news followed. In February 1990, the PRO and its data manager—the daughter of the PRO's chief executive officer—were the subjects of a nine-count criminal indictment by a Florida grand jury for fraud and making false statements. The charges against the data manager carried a maximum of $1.75 million in fines and 35 years in prison. The criminal charges against the PRO carried a maximum fine of $4.5 million. The CEO herself was named in the criminal suit, but was not indicted.

The California PRO is generally accessible through its lawyers, but the Florida PRO rarely answers questions about its legal problems. For months its only public rebuttal consisted of a three-page press release that denied the charges made in the criminal indict-

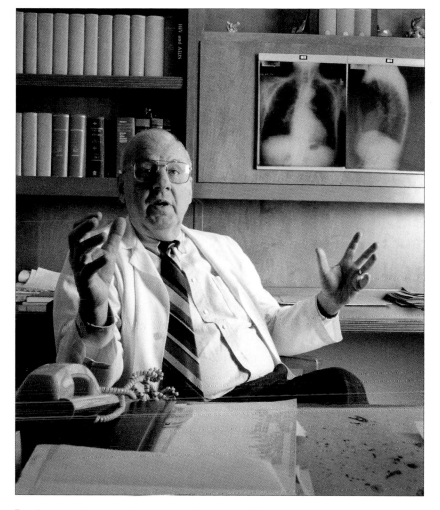

Dr. Laurie Dozier alleged the Florida PRO denied a payment and sent a letter to his patient only two days after Dr. Dozier had criticized the agency in a meeting. He sued and won, but the PRO has appealed.

ment but made no mention of the indicted data manager. In the late fall of 1990, a Florida PRO attorney finally did comment, calling the criminal case "a stupid prosecution" and vowing that the PRO and the data manager would be exonerated in a jury trial, scheduled to take place in February 1991 in the Tampa federal court. The Florida PRO had no intention of settling out of court, the attorney said.

That fraud case isn't the only damaging court action the Florida PRO has encountered. In the fall of 1989, a federal jury awarded $360,000 to a Florida internist after he claimed that actions of the Florida PRO had damaged his reputation.

Dr. Laurie Dozier, a 63-year-old board-certified internist, claimed that in September 1986, two days after he and two colleagues at Tallahassee Memorial Regional Medical Center had criticized PRO operations during a meeting with a PRO physician, the PRO denied payment for a heart patient Dr. Dozier had treated. The denial letter, sent over the signature of the PRO's medical director, stated that Dr. Dozier's treatment was unsatisfactory and that the "quality of care given on previous admission was inadequate, requiring second admission."

There were problems with the letter. First, it was sent before the physician had been given the opportunity to rebut the charges, which contravenes federal review policy. (The opportunity to rebut was given upon appeal, and the PRO overruled itself and allowed the payment). Second, it was sent not only to the doctor but to the hospital's administrator, its billing office, and the chairman of its utilization-review committee, thus exposing the physician's reputation to damage. Third, and most important, it was sent to Dr. Dozier's patient. Sending the letter to the patient, said the suit, filed in summer 1987, was "in violation of internal and federal regulations [and] was motivated by ill will, hostility, and an evil intention to defame and injure" Dr. Dozier for having dared to criticize PRO operations.

The Florida PRO's attorneys countered that the whole affair was caused not by ill will, but by a complicated clerical error. They claimed a secretary had signed the medical director's name on the letter, had independently entered the damaging language from a chart abstract, and had inadvertently sent the letter to Dr. Dozier's patient. Dr. Dozier's attorney, charging that all three of the physicians who had criticized the PRO at the hospital meeting had received denial notices shortly thereafter, called that a "series of remarkable coincidences."

"You can't use the 'My girl [the secretary] did it' defense as a PRO any better than a physician can," said attorney Alice Gosfield, noting that when the tables are turned, physicians and other providers are held accountable for their documentation in PRO disputes. The PRO's argument is nothing more than an evasion, Gosfield added: "It's outrageous that they would say that."

In October 1989, a federal jury in Tallahassee directed the PRO to pay Dr. Dozier $100,000 in compensatory damages and $250,000 in punitive damages. The jury also ordered the PRO's medical director—over whose signature the letter had been sent—to pay $10,000 in punitive damages.

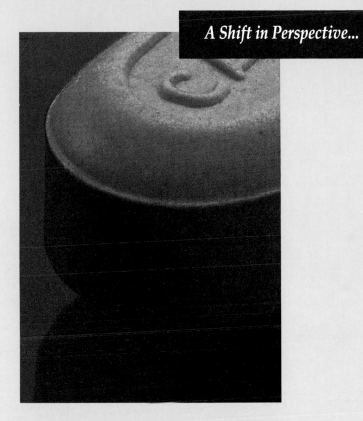

Knowing Where We Are Today...

A Shift in Perspective Makes a World of Difference

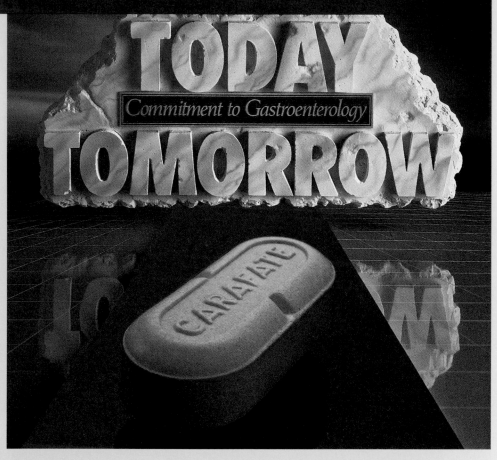

Knowing Where We Are Today...
We Set a Course For Tomorrow

With a line of GI products which, in addition to CARAFATE® (sucralfate), includes BENTYL® (dicyclomine HCl), CANTIL® (mepenzolate bromide), CHRONULAC® (lactulose), CITRUCEL®, and GAVISCON®, Marion Merrell Dow builds on the past and looks to the future with hope and enthusiasm. We're currently conducting extensive research in the areas of esophagitis, ulcerative colitis, and Crohn's disease. Through such research and through a wide range of programs and services, we offer a world of support for Gastroenterology. It's a long-term commitment; we know where we're going.

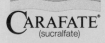

CARAFATE®
(sucralfate)

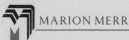

MARION MERRELL DOW INC.

The trial judge later reduced the total award to $150,000, and the government has appealed on behalf of the PRO, but the case unquestionably has further damaged the Florida PRO's reputation.

Cases like Dr. Dozier's, in which a local PRO apparently retaliates against providers who criticize them, are rare. Nonetheless, they are not unheard of. Attorney Gosfield says physicians who suspect they may be victims of such an action should call their personal lawyers or file a contract compliance complaint with HCFA's central office in Baltimore, which is responsible for the performance of PRO contractors.

Throughout the legal wrangling in both Florida and California, HCFA's PRO chief, Thomas Morford, has said little in public except that both PROs are "innocent until proven guilty." The California PRO has made much of the fact that HCFA renewed its contract the same month the civil suit was unsealed, substantially boosting the PRO's compensation in the process. The PRO's supporters argue that HCFA had word of what was coming and renewed the contract, worth $83 million through March 31, 1992, as a vote of confidence. HCFA officials note that it includes an escape clause permitting termination upon specific findings of law, and they argue that this clause was the only positive action the agency needed to take against the contractor because the PRO had not been accused of criminal actions and because Snodgrass—the employee who was—had departed.

The three-year, $49 million Florida PRO contract, which also runs through March 31, 1992, had been renewed well before the whistle-blower allegations surfaced. But because that PRO faced criminal charges, HCFA quietly sent a senior official to inspect the group's operations. The official stayed only a few days and reported that the group appeared to be operating in compliance with the law and its contract, and emergency action was not warranted.

Some in Washington, including officials who work for HHS inspector general Kusserow, think HCFA has been less vigilant than it should have been in overseeing the PROs. While it's hard to see how a program manager in Baltimore or Atlanta could have known about a mere 212 denial decisions at the Florida PRO (which reviews as many as 10,000 inpatient records a month), the dimensions of the California case are much greater. Here the PRO is accused of failing to conduct more than 50,000 reviews. PROs are contractually obligated to report monthly review results to regional operations managers. If an extraordinarily high number of cases was reviewed in just a few days, as the whistle-blowers suggest, why didn't the regional manager notice it? Or if he did, why didn't any federal officials question the PRO's behavior? Much about the California case remains unknown, and may never be known publicly because the PRO speaks only through its attorneys. HCFA officials are reluctant to speak on the record. Off the record, federal officials who refuse to be named acknowledge having serious misgivings about the PROs' behavior. Only time will tell whether those misgivings are justified; meanwhile, the 52 PROs that have never been charged with serious wrongdoing continue to operate in what must be assumed to be an honest manner.

CHAPTER EIGHT

THE FUTURE

T he controversy surrounding PROs continued to rage on all sides as the program entered the 1990s. Early in 1990, a blue-ribbon panel assembled by the prestigious Institute of Medicine (IOM) in Washington announced the results of a two-year, $1.7 million study (*Medicare: A Strategy for Quality Assurance*) that was so critical of the PRO system it immediately inspired wide debate.

Formed by congressional mandate, its 17 members representing the whole spectrum of groups concerned with health care, the committee argued that the PRO effort is misguided. Its focus on punitive actions against a handful of aberrant providers, said the study, prevents it from pursuing goals that might have a lasting and positive influence on mainstream medicine. Moreover, says the two-volume report, the PRO system doesn't measure Medicare's effects on patients.

Even while agreeing with some of the study's conclusions, HCFA defended its program and put forth the Universal Clinical Data Set system as a way to placate critics.

The IOM report gives considerable space to doctors' criticisms of PROs: "Many physicians remain suspicious of and hostile to PRO activities, continuing to perceive it [*sic*] at one and the same time as intrusive, arbitrary and punitive, and fundamentally irrelevant to improving quality of care." One committee member, Monsignor Charles Fahey, a professor of aging studies at Fordham University, even accused the PRO program of "infantilizing" providers.

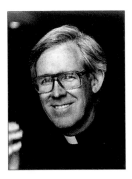

Monsignor Charles Fahey: PROs "infantilize" providers.

The study recommends replacing the PROs with a system fostering "continuous quality improvement," a concept most commonly associated with industrial quality-control techniques. This approach, say its backers, relies on workers' professionalism and ability to internalize precepts, and gives employees a personal stake in their organization's commitment to change. Under the proposed plan, hospitals and other providers (as opposed to federal bureaucrats) would devise their own qualilty-control systems, and cost containment would be eliminated as an objective. The proposed groups, called Medicare quality review organizations (MQROs) in the study, would replace PROs in three phases over 10 years. External organizations would be responsible only for analyzing broad patterns of treatment, intervening when institutions were unwilling or unable to exercise their responsibilities, and for examining Medicare's long-term effects on the health of the elderly.

Although the IOM panel plainly viewed the PRO program as a relic, it conceded that continuous quality improvement has yet to be tested nationally in the context of the practice of medicine. "Whether health-care institutions and facilities can successfully implement the continuous improvement approach with a focus on meaningful medical, nursing, and other professional quality-of-care issues will have to be tested rigorously over the next few years," it concluded.

HCFA, in a classically turf-conscious response, said it supported the bulk of the IOM's recommendations but objected to the panel's call for a commission of outside overseers and a national council to guide MQRO implementation. And despite her advocacy of internal quality measures, HCFA administrator Gail Wilensky said that the IOM study underestimated the need to detect aberrant providers, and she opposed IOM's call for doubling Medicare quality-assurance funding. She called the panel's cost estimates "not very convincing."

More important, HCFA proceeded to rally around the Uniform Clinical Data Set, its automated, interactive system for screening care, which is still unfinished. The subject of unusually secretive pilot testing since 1987 by the Wisconsin PRO and researchers at Queen's University in Toronto, UCDS is intended to standardize PRO case screenings. Under this system, all PRO nurses and records technicians use computerized algorithms that incorporate about 1,600 clinical data elements to screen records for inappropriate or poor-quality care. Operating correctly, UCDS is supposed to ensure that PRO nurses in New Mexico and Vermont would refer the same cases for review at roughly the same rate. (As now, only PRO physicians would be able to act against another physician or an institution.) Proponents believe UCDS will also permit HCFA to build a huge database of clinical information that will enable it to compare usage rates between regions of the country and to generate statistics indicating which treatments work best for which groups of patients.

Citing as an example the several hundred thousand diabetics admitted to U.S. hospitals annually, Dr. Thomas Dehn, the former AMPRA president, says, "Using UCDS, we'll be able to figure out what's the single best way to treat an uncontrolled diabetic on admission. It's an incredible opportunity for medicine to take a step forward in terms of quality and efficiency."

PROs in Alabama, Arizona, Colorado, Connecticut, Iowa, Utah, and Wisconsin were scheduled to begin making on-line case referrals using UCDS early in 1991. Another dozen or so states are to begin using the system in April 1992. All PROs are expected to be using it within a couple of years after that.

UCDS isn't perfect. Pilot testing has so far revealed problems with "false positives"—cases that are referred when they should not have been—as well as with "false negatives"—cases that should have been referred but weren't. Worse, say experts, nurses using UCDS have been referring about 50 percent of all cases reviewed to doctors for further review, whereas the current system's rate is 20 to 40 percent. Since HCFA has decreed that UCDS will be budget-neutral (its total costs cannot exceed the cost of the current PRO program), it must either lower the UCDS referral rate or reduce the total number of cases reviewed. If UCDS continues to compel nurses to refer nearly half the cases they abstract, HCFA might be forced to cut screening to no more than 10 percent of all Medicare admissions. Though this would render U.S. hospitals less vulnerable to Medicare payment denials, consumers and outside researchers would surely ask whether review of only 10 percent of admissions is enough to guarantee quality of care.

Another operational problem concerns the time needed to do reviews: HCFA concedes that the automated system allows abstracters to complete only five cases per day, as opposed to 10 to 15 currently. Again, if HCFA is to hold total costs constant, the number of reviews conducted will be even lower than now.

Critics of UCDS abound. Dr. Dennis O'Leary, chief of the Joint Commission on Accreditation of Healthcare Organizations, argues that UCDS, far from promoting a quality-assurance system that allows providers to find local solutions to local problems, is nothing but a more ingenious external screening system.

"I don't think it's established that UCDS provides a more useful screening mechanism than the current system," says Dr. O'Leary. Even if it did, he says, the same old preoccupation with what he variously describes as "scalp hunting" and a "get-the-bastards mentality" is still there. "HCFA's narrow view would seem to be that the same agency is supposed to do all this monitoring and quality-of-care promotion," he complains. "What's missing in this system is the possibility for networking. No one talks to one another."

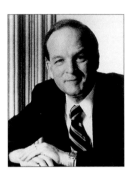

Dr. Dennis O'Leary, JCAHO chief and UCDS critic.

Other experts are even more withering about UCDS, at least in private. One insider claims UCDS will be prohibitively expensive and that the scientific validity of the computer program used to run it is questionable. The critic suggests that before they do anything else, the anonymous architects of the system should describe in a credible scientific journal the methodology they used. "I think it's just going to be a terrible mistake," he continues. "Once evaluation is done, the emperor's lack of clothes will become manifest."

"It has all the makings of a Gallipoli," says another critic with a close working knowledge of the project.

Katherine Lohr of the Institute of Medicine argues that with UCDS, HCFA is overlooking key concepts of the IOM report, such as the need for consensus building, for gathering quality-of-life information from patients, and for expanding quality review into important non-hospital settings like physicians' offices and home health agencies.

The Health Standards and Quality Bureau responds that it does intend to disclose the clinical indicators from which UCDS's computerized algorithms were derived; that UCDS will once and for all ensure that the right cases are referred to physician-advisers; and that ultimately the new system represents a leap forward in meeting the much-discussed need to measure clinical outcomes, as opposed to mere processes. HSQB chief Morford accuses his critics of professional jealousy. He thinks Dr. O'Leary, Lohr, and the rest know the UCDS train is leaving the station but are having a hard time deciding whether or not to board.

Other HSQB officials aren't so optimistic. One has told colleagues privately that UCDS is a major undertaking for a staff already stretched to the limit and that the mechanics of the system have proved daunting. The same person says HCFA has had difficulty just getting the staff time needed to make relatively simple adjustments to the computer program.

Even as UCDS goes forward, the PRO issue that generates the most emotion among physicians right now is office-based review. Rather cavalierly mandated by Congress as just one of the expansions of review authority into ambulatory settings in 1986, PRO review of Medicare records from physicians' private offices impresses quite a few doctors as the Orwellian nightmare made manifest. The mere prospect has led some to conjure the image of PRO bureaucrats rampaging through offices, interrogating patients, and generally wreaking havoc. When HCFA launched a two-year, seven-state, $2.7 million pilot project led by the Wisconsin PRO and the Medical College of Wisconsin in 1990, Dr. Grant Rodkey, chairman of the AMA Council on Medical Service, said the enterprise was akin to "having the Gestapo in your front room." The remark embarrassed cooler heads at the AMA, and HCFA was furious. Dr. Rodkey himself later conceded he'd been impolitic. Still, there's no getting around the obvious: many physicians feel that review of private office records crosses the line that separates legitimate peer review from state-sponsored harassment.

Morford and HCFA, careful to note that the idea came from Congress, have approved only modest pilot projects in which physicians' participation is voluntary and no financial penalties are imposed. The Wisconsin project—which includes PROs in Arizona, Connecticut, Indiana, North Carolina, Utah, and Washington—is advertised as an educational program focusing on 16 conditions commonly treated in private offices. Questioned cases, say program planners, are reviewed only by board-certified or board-eligible specialists. A second pilot, led by the Maryland PRO and researchers from Harvard University, Johns Hopkins, and Park Nicollet Medical Foundation, began in September 1990 and has been given $2.9 million for three years. It concentrates on internists and general practitioners, and physicians who choose to participate receive confidential reports comparing their performance with that of anonymous peers. Leaders of both projects emphasize that PRO reviewers do not visit physicians' offices—chart reviews are handled by mail. HCFA has the power to order office-based review nationally, but has so far chosen not to do so. The agency may be waiting to see whether the pilot projects prove workable. If not, HCFA always has the option of going back to Congress and advocating repeal or revision.

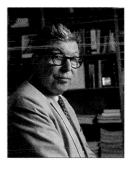

Dr. Grant Rodkey of the AMA likened office-based review to Gestapo tactics.

Meanwhile, it seems that organized medicine has at least tacitly decided that the PROs are here to stay. Despite rhetoric to the contrary, leaders of state medical societies are working closely with PROs, and in some cases running them. In the fall of 1990, the AMA won a competitive bid to function as HCFA's "physician consultant" in arbitrating clinical review disputes between PROs and the super-PRO. Under a modest one-year agreement, renewable for four additional years, the leading voice of organized medicine now reviews and adjudicates disputes over payment denials and adverse quality determinations.

The long-term implications of that contract are significant. First, it's likely to become increasingly difficult for the AMA's rank-and-file members to throw stones at PROs once they see that the association is directly involved in PRO management. Second, the AMA has indicated it will solicit the help of state and specialty societies in finding physicians to participate as reviewers, thus further eroding the distinction between the reviewers and the reviewed. Finally, by the very nature of the contract, AMA will have to take sides. Few doubt that the AMA will side with local review doctors who are duty-bound to consult with attending physicians before they act, rather than with the superPRO, which is not. In short order, the AMA could find itself converted from the PROs' chief antagonist to their chief ally.

Would that be a bad thing? Despite the accusations of the more vociferous elements of organized medicine, PROs today are locally organized groups of active-practice colleagues who attend meetings voluntarily and thrash out difficult issues that get to the heart of how medicine polices itself. To be sure, there are plenty of faceless bureaucrats in Washington and Baltimore; there are doubtless plenty of tough-minded CEOs making sure PRO employees fill work quotas. But none of these people has even indirect authority to deny a single hospital payment, demand that a physician undergo remedial education, or recommend that he or she be expelled from Medicare. Federal law is unambiguous: those powers reside exclusively with physicians. Thus, although certain antagonisms are built in to the process, PROs are only as aggressive or passive as physicians want them to be.

Of course, if Congress were to conclude that the program has evolved into nothing more than an elaborate form of window-dressing, it could change the law, and physicians could lose that authority. But no such conclusion has been reached—Congress keeps giving more authority to PROs, not less. And even as budget pressures invite more and more tinkering with reimbursement formulas, the program will continue to be viewed as a way to ensure uncompromised care for the nation's more than 30 million Medicare beneficiaries. That is supposedly the end that PROs exist to

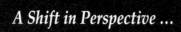

A Shift in Perspective ...

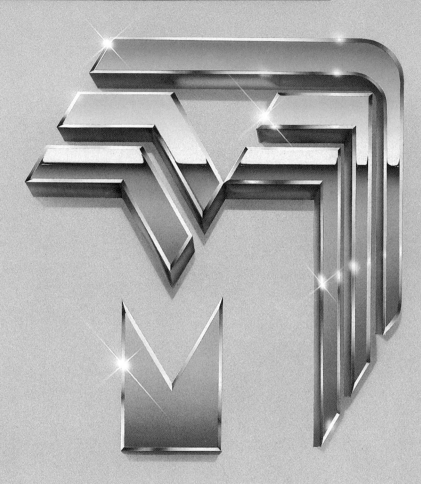

The combining of two entities–Marion Laboratories and Merrell Dow Pharmaceuticals, each with its own distinctive personality and singular strengths–was a result of being open to new perspectives...new worlds of possibility. Marion Merrell Dow is greater than the sum of its parts, an innovative company devoted to quality... committed to research...responsible for providing a safe and healthy workplace... mindful of the environment...and respectful of our associates, suppliers, and customers. Our only unalterable perspective is the awareness that the ultimate beneficiary of all our efforts is the ultimate user of our products, the patient.

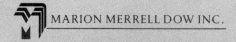

MARION MERRELL DOW INC.

further, and it would be difficult to find anyone who opposes it. The furor over PROs came about and continues solely because of disagreement by various interest groups about the means chosen to achieve that end.

Former HCFA administrator William Roper, now director of the Centers for Disease Control in Atlanta, recalls a comprehensive review of the PRO program he undertook in the summer of 1986 in which consumer, provider, and physician leaders were asked to offer their views on the future of PROs.

"My conclusion, and the department's conclusion," says Dr. Roper, "was that if we didn't have the program, we'd invent something a lot like it."

GLOSSARY

AMPRA: The American Medical Peer Review Association, a trade group that represents PROs in Washington (see Chapter 4).

Appropriateness review: PRO retrospective reviews of hospital admissions. Payment denials are predicated on lack of medical necessity.

DRGs: Diagnosis related groups, a classification system Medicare uses to cluster illnesses into more than 400 groups of like diagnoses, each labeled with a code number. Under the Prospective Payment System (PPS), Medicare reimburses costs according to the DRG assignment. PROs audit selected hospital records to ensure that DRG coding is correct (see Chapter 4).

Generic quality screens: Written medical criteria in the form of checklists that PRO nurse-reviewers compare against each medical record under review. Generic quality screens are designed to detect the possibility of poor quality of care. Criteria vary according to the site where medical care was rendered (hospital, nursing home, home health agency). Cases that fail screens are referred to PRO physician-advisers for review (see Chapter 5).

HCFA: The U.S. Health Care Financing Administration, the agency within the federal Department of Health and Human Services that has overall responsibility for management of the PRO program. Its headquarters are in Baltimore. Regional managers operate 10 offices in major cities throughout the United States (see Chapter 3).

HSQB: The Health Standards and Quality Bureau of HCFA. It manages the day-to-day operation of the PRO program (see Chapter 3).

Inspector general (IG) of the Department of Health and Human Services: A presidential appointee who has watchdog power over physicians. The IG's office approves sanction recommendations PROs make against physicians or other providers (see chapters 3 and 4).

Institute of Medicine (IOM): The Washington, D.C., health-policy and research center that is affiliated with the National Academy of Sciences. Its 1990 study of Medicare quality assurance advocates a total revamping of the PRO program. With a membership that includes leading physicians and health-care-policy analysts, IOM frequently advises Congress and the federal government on key policy issues (see Chapter 8).

PPS: The Medicare Prospective Payment System, which reimburses hospital costs on the basis of payments fixed in advance by the DRG system. The imposition of PPS beginning in 1983 caused the PRO program to shift its emphasis from utilization review to quality review (see Chapter 1).

Preprocedure review: Authorization by telephone of 10 elective surgical procedures before the procedures take place. Medicare requires prior approval of all cataract and carotid endarterectomy surgeries, as well as eight more procedures that PROs may choose from a list provided by HCFA (see Appendix).

QIP: The Quality Intervention Plan, a PRO system instituted with the third scope of work in 1988. A weighted point system, the QIP requires PROs to intervene in specific ways when a physician accumulates a certain number of quality-of-care demerits on his or her record (see Chapter 6).

Retrospective review: Review of certain medical records by PRO nurse-reviewers after treatment has been provided. Medicare may deny payment for all or part of the provider's services if the results of an unfavorable review are upheld by a PRO physician-adviser (see Appendix).

Risk-sharing HMOs: Health maintenance organizations that enroll Medicare beneficiaries in exchange for a predetermined flat rate per patient per month (called capitation). This puts the HMO at financial risk because it must cover treatment costs in excess of the monthly capitation rates. HMOs may keep money they do not expend for patient care. PROs review all risk-sharing HMOs for quality of care (see Appendix).

Sanctions: Medicare fines or exclusions of physicians or other providers levied on the basis of a PRO's finding that a reviewed treatment did not meet local, professionally recognized standards of care. Sanctions can be appealed, and they cannot take effect unless the physician or provider is judged "unwilling or unable" to improve (see Chapter 6).

Scope of work: The name of the document that delineates the rules under which PROs operate during a given contract period. There have been three scopes of work since the PRO program began. Now operating under the third, PROs will switch to the fourth scope of work in 1991 (see Chapter 5).

Substandard quality denials: A plan authorized by Congress in 1986 but not yet in effect that would allow PROs to routinely deny payment for provider services that do not meet professionally recognized standards of care. PROs may now deny payment only for services judged unnecessary or inappropriate (see Chapter 6).

UCDS: The Uniform Clinical Data Set, a computerized system now under development at HCFA that is intended to automate initial PRO case screenings and obtain uniform results for each case reviewed. HCFA will compile the clinical information obtained by the screening and use it to analyze practice patterns and clinical outcomes (see Chapter 8).

APPENDIX

Review Requirements: Third Scope of Work

Under the third scope of work, PROs must review the following:

■ A 3 percent random sample of discharges from each PPS hospital.

■ 50 percent of all transfers from one PPS hospital to another.

■ 100 percent of transfers from standard to psychiatric beds when billing records fail to show valid ICD-9-CM codes; 100 percent of records showing organic brain conditions; and a 10 percent random sample of the remaining transfers from a PPS to a non-PPS bed in the same hospital.

■ 25 percent of transfers from PPS "swing" beds in the same hospital.

■ A random 25 percent hospital-specific sample of all PPS hospital readmissions within 31 days of discharge (review of both stays).

■ "Intervening care" when provided for at least 20 percent of patients readmitted to a particular hospital. (This care is defined as occurring between admission and readmission and delivered by a skilled nursing facility, home health agency, or hospital outpatient department.)

■ DRGs viewed as having a high risk for quality problems and/or miscoding:
(a) 25 percent of cases coded as DRG 462 (rehabilitation)
(b) 50 percent of DRG 468 (unrelated OR procedures)
(c) 100 percent of DRG 385 (neonates, died or transferred)
(d) 100 percent of DRG 386 (neonates, extreme immaturity)
(e) 100 percent of DRG 387 (prematurity with major problems)
(f) 100 percent of DRG 388 (prematurity without major problems)

(g) 100 percent of DRG 389 (full-term neonate with major problems)

(h) 100 percent of DRG 390 (neonate with other significant problems)

(i) 100 percent of DRG 391 (normal newborn)

(j) 100 percent of DRG 472 (extensive burns)

(k) 100 percent of DRG 474 (tracheostomy)

(l) 100 percent of DRG 475 (mechanical ventilation through endotracheal intubation).

■ A 25 percent random sample of day and cost outliers (focusing on cases with billed charges $3,000 or more above cost outlier threshold).

■ Postpayment review of all cases with the following principal diagnoses:

(a) Diabetes mellitus, without mention of complication, non-insulin-dependent

(b) Diabetes mellitus, without mention of complication, insulin-dependent

(c) Obesity

(d) Impacted cerumen

(e) Benign hypertension

(f) Left bundle branch hemiblock

(g) Other left bundle branch block

(h) Right bundle branch block

(i) Positive SRL/VRL HL3

(j) Elevated blood pressure reading without diagnosis of hypertension

(k) Other and unspecified complication of medical care, not elsewhere specified

(l) Cardiac pacemaker (fitting and adjustment).

■ All hospital-submitted DRG claims adjustments resulting in higher-weighted DRGs.

■ All cases in which the hospital initially determined the admission wasn't covered but subsequently the patient required a covered level of care.

■ Cases forwarded by the fiscal intermediaries that process Part A claims seeking a determination of medical necessity; cases forwarded by HCFA regional offices in instances when skilled nursing-facility care is viewed as insufficient, raising the possibility of premature discharge from a hospital.

■ A 15 percent random sample of discharges from a PPS bed to PPS-exempt unit in the same hospital; review of a 15 percent random sample of discharges from PPS-exempt hospital units in which patients had been admitted from home or another institution.

■ A 15 percent random sample of discharges from PPS-exempt hospitals in which the patient is admitted directly or transferred from another hospital.

■ A 5 percent random sample of all surgical cases from ambulatory-surgery centers and hospital outpatient areas (excluding cataract surgeries).

■ 100 percent preprocedure review of 10 elective procedures, including cataract extractions (except when performed in physicians' private offices) and carotid endarterectomies (even if the procedure isn't part of a principal diagnosis); PROs choose eight other procedures from a list of 11 provided by HCFA, including prostatectomy, pacemaker implantation and reimplantation, cholecystectomy (total or partial), inguinal hernia, laminectomy, complex peripheral revascularization, coronary artery bypass with graft, major joint replacement (hip or knee), percutaneous transluminal coronary angioplasty, bunionectomy, and hysterectomy; quarterly postprocedure review of a sample of cases to ensure appropriateness of prior approvals; retrospective review of emergency surgeries.

■ 100 percent preprocedure review when cataract surgeons request the use of assistants.

■ Cardiac catheterization when requested by insurance companies processing Medicare Part B claims for HCFA.

■ 100 percent of hospital-issued notices of noncoverage to beneficiaries when the physician disagrees with the hospital and the hospital requests a review; 100 percent of cases in which the patient disputes the hospital's notice; 100 percent of cases in which the patient is liable for charges occurring after notification by hospital; 100 percent of cases in which the hospital determined the admission wasn't covered.

■ All written complaints from beneficiaries and their representatives concerning quality of care, assuming services were covered by Medicare and provided in Medicare-certified facilities.

■ Three months' worth of cases from physicians identified by state medical boards as having had disciplinary actions taken against them— excluding review of cases drawn from physicians' private offices.

■ Inpatient, ambulatory, and posthospital services provided to beneficiaries enrolled in HMOs that participate in Medicare on a "risk-sharing" basis; review of 13 conditions in all settings; review of a 3 percent sample of inpatient cases; review of ambulatory care; review of nontraumatic deaths in all settings; review of transfers and readmissions from hospitals.

■ All suspected "patient dumping" incidents referred by HCFA.

■ All cases where a hospital determined that an admission was not covered and the patient required a covered level of care later in the stay.

Additional Copies

To order additional copies of *The Doctor Watchers*
for friends or colleagues, please write to The Grand
Rounds Press, Whittle Direct Books, 505 Market St.,
Knoxville, Tenn. 37902. Please include the recipient's
name, mailing address, and, where applicable, primary
specialty and ME number.

For a single copy, please enclose a check for $21.95
plus $1.50 for postage and handling, payable to The
Grand Rounds Press. When ordering 10 or more books,
enclose $20.95 for each plus $5 for postage and
handling; for orders of 50 or more books, enclose
$19.95 for each plus $20 for postage and handling. For
more information about The Grand Rounds Press,
please call 800-765-5889.

Please allow four weeks for delivery.
Tennessee residents must add 7¾ percent sales tax.

Professional Use Information

CARDIZEM®

(diltiazem HCl) Tablets

DESCRIPTION

CARDIZEM® (diltiazem hydrochloride) is a calcium ion influx inhibitor (slow channel blocker or calcium antagonist). Chemically, diltiazem hydrochloride is 1,5-Benzothiazepin-4(5H)one,3-(acetyloxy)-5-[2-(dimethylamino)ethyl]-2,3-dihydro-2-(4-methoxyphenyl)-, monohydrochloride, (+) -cis-. The chemical structure is:

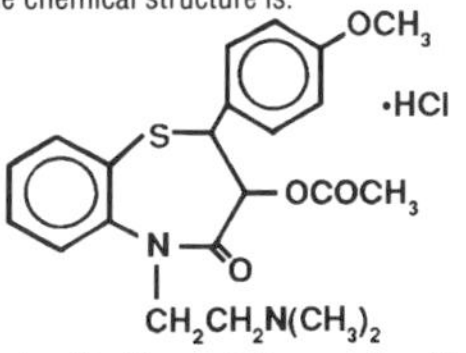

Diltiazem hydrochloride is a white to off-white crystalline powder with a bitter taste. It is soluble in water, methanol, and chloroform. It has a molecular weight of 450.98. Each tablet of CARDIZEM contains 30 mg, 60 mg, 90 mg, or 120 mg diltiazem hydrochloride.

Also contains: D&C Yellow #10, FD&C Yellow #6 (60 mg and 120 mg), or FD&C Blue #1 (30 mg and 90 mg), hydroxypropylcellulose, hydroxypropyl methylcellulose, lactose, magnesium stearate, methylparaben, polyethylene glycol, talc, and other ingredients.

For oral administration.

CLINICAL PHARMACOLOGY

The therapeutic benefits achieved with CARDIZEM are believed to be related to its ability to inhibit the influx of calcium ions during membrane depolarization of cardiac and vascular smooth muscle.

Mechanisms of Action. Although precise mechanisms of its antianginal actions are still being delineated, CARDIZEM is believed to act in the following ways:

1. Angina Due to Coronary Artery Spasm: CARDIZEM has been shown to be a potent dilator of coronary arteries both epicardial and subendocardial. Spontaneous and ergonovine-induced coronary artery spasm are inhibited by CARDIZEM.
2. Exertional Angina: CARDIZEM has been shown to produce increases in exercise tolerance, probably due to its ability to reduce myocardial oxygen demand. This is accomplished via reductions in heart rate and systemic blood pressure at submaximal and maximal exercise work loads.

In animal models, diltiazem interferes with the slow inward (depolarizing) current in excitable tissue. It causes excitation-contraction uncoupling in various myocardial tissues without changes in the configuration of the action potential. Diltiazem produces relaxation of coronary vascular smooth muscle and dilation of both large and small coronary arteries at drug levels which cause little or no negative inotropic effect. The resultant increases in coronary blood flow (epicardial and subendocardial) occur in ischemic and nonischemic models and are accompanied by dose-dependent decreases in systemic blood pressure and decreases in peripheral resistance.

Hemodynamic and Electrophysiologic Effects. Like other calcium antagonists, diltiazem decreases sinoatrial and atrioventricular conduction in isolated tissues and has a negative inotropic effect in isolated preparations. In the intact animal, prolongation of the AH interval can be seen at higher doses.

In man, diltiazem prevents spontaneous and ergonovine-provoked coronary artery spasm. It causes a decrease in peripheral vascular resistance and a modest fall in blood pressure and, in exercise tolerance studies in patients with ischemic heart disease, reduces the heart rate-blood pressure product for any given work load. Studies to date, primarily in patients with good ventricular function, have not revealed evidence of a negative inotropic effect; cardiac output, ejection fraction, and left ventricular end diastolic pressure have not been affected. There are as yet few data on the interaction of diltiazem and beta-blockers. Resting heart rate is usually unchanged or slightly reduced by diltiazem.

Intravenous diltiazem in doses of 20 mg prolongs AH conduction time and AV node functional and effective refractory periods approximately 20%. In a study involving single oral doses of 300 mg of CARDIZEM in six normal volunteers, the average maximum PR prolongation was 14% with no instances of greater than first-degree AV block. Diltiazem-associated prolongation of the AH interval is not more pronounced in patients with first-degree heart block. In patients with sick sinus syndrome, diltiazem significantly prolongs sinus cycle length (up to 50% in some cases).

Chronic oral administration of CARDIZEM in doses of up to 240 mg/day has resulted in small increases in PR interval, but has not usually produced abnormal prolongation.

Pharmacokinetics and Metabolism. Diltiazem is absorbed from the tablet formulation to about 80% of a reference capsule and is subject to an extensive first-pass effect, giving an absolute bioavailability (compared to intravenous dosing) of about 40%. CARDIZEM undergoes extensive hepatic metabolism in which 2% to 4% of the unchanged drug appears in the urine. In vitro binding studies show CARDIZEM is 70% to 80% bound to plasma proteins. Competitive ligand binding studies have also shown CARDIZEM binding is not altered by therapeutic concentrations of digoxin, hydrochlorothiazide, phenylbutazone, propranolol, salicylic acid, or warfarin. Single oral doses of 30 to 120 mg of CARDIZEM result in detectable plasma levels within 30 to 60 minutes and peak plasma levels two to three hours after drug administration. The plasma elimination half-life following single or multiple drug administration is approximately 3.5 hours. Desacetyl diltiazem is also present in the plasma at levels of 10% to 20% of the parent drug and is 25% to 50% as potent as a coronary vasodilator as diltiazem. Therapeutic blood levels of CARDIZEM appear to be in the range of 50-200 ng/mL. There is a departure from dose-linearity when single doses above 60 mg are given; a 120-mg dose gave blood levels three times that of the 60-mg dose. There is no information about the effect of renal or hepatic impairment on excretion or metabolism of diltiazem.

INDICATIONS AND USAGE

1. **Angina Pectoris Due to Coronary Artery Spasm.** CARDIZEM is indicated in the treatment of angina pectoris due to coronary artery spasm. CARDIZEM has been shown effective in the treatment of spontaneous coronary artery spasm presenting as Prinzmetal's variant angina (resting angina with ST-segment elevation occurring during attacks).
2. **Chronic Stable Angina (Classic Effort-Associated Angina).** CARDIZEM is indicated in the management of chronic stable angina in patients who cannot tolerate therapy with beta-blockers and/or nitrates or who remain symptomatic despite adequate doses of these agents. CARDIZEM has been effective in short-term controlled trials in reducing angina frequency and increasing exercise tolerance but confirmation of sustained effectiveness is incomplete.

There are few controlled studies of the effectiveness of the concomitant use of diltiazem and beta-blockers or of the safety of this combination in patients with impaired ventricular function or conduction abnormalities.

CONTRAINDICATIONS

CARDIZEM is contraindicated in (1) patients with sick sinus syndrome except in the presence of a functioning ventricular pacemaker, (2) patients with second- or third-degree AV block except in the presence of a functioning ventricular pacemaker, (3) patients with hypotension (less than 90 mm Hg systolic), (4) patients who have demonstrated hypersensitivity to the drug, and (5) patients with acute myocardial infarction and pulmonary congestion documented by x-ray on admission.

WARNINGS

1. **Cardiac Conduction.** CARDIZEM prolongs AV node refractory periods without significantly prolonging sinus node recovery time, except in patients with sick sinus syndrome. This effect may rarely result in abnormally slow heart rates (particularly in patients with sick sinus syndrome) or second- or third-degree AV block (six of 1,243 patients for 0.48%). Concomitant use of diltiazem with beta-blockers or digitalis may result in additive effects on cardiac conduction. A patient with Prinzmetal's angina developed periods of asystole (2 to 5 seconds) after a single dose of 60 mg of diltiazem.
2. **Congestive Heart Failure.** Although diltiazem has a negative inotropic effect in isolated animal tissue preparations, hemodynamic studies in humans with normal ventricular function have not shown a reduction in cardiac index nor consistent negative effects on contractility (dp/dt). Experience with the use of CARDIZEM alone or in combination with beta-blockers in patients with impaired ventricular function is very limited. Caution should be exercised when using the drug in such patients.
3. **Hypotension.** Decreases in blood pressure associated with CARDIZEM therapy may occasionally result in symptomatic hypotension.
4. **Acute Hepatic Injury.** In rare instances, significant elevations in enzymes such as alkaline phosphatase, LDH, SGOT, SGPT, and other phenomena consistent with acute hepatic injury have been noted. These reactions have been reversible upon discontinuation of drug therapy. The relationship to CARDIZEM is uncertain in most cases, but probable in some. (See PRECAUTIONS.)

PRECAUTIONS

General. CARDIZEM (diltiazem hydrochloride) is extensively metabolized by the liver and excreted by the kidneys and in bile. As with any drug given over prolonged periods, laboratory parameters should be monitored at regular intervals. The drug should be used with caution in patients with impaired renal or hepatic function. In subacute and chronic dog and rat studies designed to produce toxicity, high doses of diltiazem were associated with hepatic damage. In special subacute hepatic studies, oral doses of 125 mg/kg and higher in rats were associated with histological changes in the liver which were reversible when the drug was discontinued. In dogs, doses of 20 mg/kg were also associated with hepatic changes, however, these changes were reversible with continued dosing.

Dermatological events (see ADVERSE REACTIONS section) may be transient and may disappear despite continued use of CARDIZEM. However, skin eruptions progressing to erythema multiforme and/or exfoliative dermatitis have also been infrequently reported. Should a dermatologic reaction persist, the drug should be discontinued.

Drug Interaction. Due to the potential for additive effects, caution and careful titration are warranted in patients receiving CARDIZEM concomitantly with any agents known to affect cardiac contractility and/or conduction. (See WARNINGS.)

Pharmacologic studies indicate that there may be additive effects in prolonging AV conduction when using beta-blockers or digitalis concomitantly with CARDIZEM. (See WARNINGS.)

As with all drugs, care should be exercised when treating patients with multiple medications. CARDIZEM undergoes biotransformation by cytochrome P-450 mixed function oxidase. Coadministration of CARDIZEM with other agents which follow the same route of biotransformation may result in the competitive inhibition of metabolism. Dosages of similarly metabolized drugs, particularly those of low therapeutic ratio or in patients with renal and/or hepatic impairment, may require adjustment when starting or stopping concomitantly administered CARDIZEM to maintain optimum therapeutic blood levels.

Beta-blockers: Controlled and uncontrolled domestic studies suggest that concomitant use of CARDIZEM and beta-blockers or digitalis is usually well tolerated. Available data are not sufficient, however, to predict the effects of concomitant treatment, particularly in patients with left ventricular dysfunction or cardiac conduction abnormalities.

Administration of CARDIZEM (diltiazem hydrochloride) concomitantly with propranolol in five normal volunteers resulted in increased propranolol levels in all subjects and bioavailability of propranolol was increased approximately 50%. If combination therapy is initiated or withdrawn in conjunction with propranolol, an adjustment in the propranolol dose may be warranted. (See WARNINGS.)

Cimetidine: A study in six healthy volunteers has shown a significant increase in peak diltiazem plasma levels (58%) and area-under-the-curve (53%) after a 1-week course of cimetidine at 1,200 mg per day and diltiazem 60 mg per day. Ranitidine produced smaller, nonsignificant increases. The effect may be mediated by cimetidine's known inhibition of hepatic cytochrome P-450, the enzyme system probably responsible for the first-pass metabolism of diltiazem. Patients currently receiving diltiazem therapy should be carefully monitored for a change in pharmacological effect when initiating and discontinuing therapy with cimetidine. An adjustment in the diltiazem dose may be warranted.

Digitalis: Administration of CARDIZEM with digoxin in 24 healthy male subjects increased plasma digoxin concentrations approximately 20%. Another investigator found no increase in digoxin levels in 12 patients with coronary artery disease. Since there have been conflicting results regarding the effect of digoxin levels, it is recommended that digoxin levels be monitored when initiating, adjusting, and discontinuing CARDIZEM therapy to avoid possible over- or under-digitalization. (See WARNINGS.)

Anesthetics: The depression of cardiac contractility, conductivity, and automaticity as well as the vascular dilation associated with anesthetics may be potentiated by calcium channel blockers. When used concomitantly, anesthetics and calcium blockers should be titrated carefully.

Carcinogenesis, Mutagenesis, Impairment of Fertility. A 24-month study in rats and a 21-month study in mice showed no evidence of carcinogenicity. There was also no mutagenic response in in vitro bacterial tests. No intrinsic effect on fertility was observed in rats.

Pregnancy. Category C. Reproduction studies have been conducted in mice, rats, and rabbits. Administration of doses ranging from five to ten times greater (on a mg/kg basis) than the daily recommended therapeutic dose has resulted in embryo and fetal lethality. These doses, in some studies, have been reported to cause skeletal abnormalities. In the perinatal/postnatal studies, there was some reduction in early individual pup weights and survival rates. There was an increased incidence of stillbirths at doses of 20 times the human dose or greater.

There are no well-controlled studies in pregnant women; therefore, use CARDIZEM in pregnant women only if the potential benefit justifies the potential risk to the fetus.

CARDIZEM®
(diltiazem HCl) Tablets

Nursing Mothers. Diltiazem is excreted in human milk. One report suggests that concentrations in breast milk may approximate serum levels. If use of CARDIZEM is deemed essential, an alternative method of infant feeding should be instituted.

Pediatric Use. Safety and effectiveness in children have not been established.

ADVERSE REACTIONS

Serious adverse reactions have been rare in studies carried out to date, but it should be recognized that patients with impaired ventricular function and cardiac conduction abnormalities have usually been excluded.

In domestic placebo-controlled trials, the incidence of adverse reactions reported during CARDIZEM therapy was not greater than that reported during placebo therapy.

The following represent occurrences observed in clinical studies which can be at least reasonably associated with the pharmacology of calcium influx inhibition. In many cases, the relationship to CARDIZEM has not been established. The most common occurrences as well as their frequency of presentation are: edema (2.4%), headache (2.1%), nausea (1.9%), dizziness (1.5%), rash (1.3%), asthenia (1.2%). In addition, the following events were reported infrequently (less than 1%):

Cardiovascular: Angina, arrhythmia, AV block (first degree), AV block (second or third degree—see conduction warning), bradycardia, congestive heart failure, flushing, hypotension, palpitations, syncope.

Nervous System: Amnesia, depression, gait abnormality, hallucinations, insomnia, nervousness, paresthesia, personality change, somnolence, tinnitus, tremor.

Gastrointestinal: Anorexia, constipation, diarrhea, dysgeusia, dyspepsia, mild elevations of alkaline phosphatase, SGOT, SGPT, and LDH (see hepatic warnings), vomiting, weight increase.

Dermatologic: Petechiae, pruritus, photosensitivity, urticaria.

Other: Amblyopia, CPK elevation, dyspnea, epistaxis, eye irritation, hyperglycemia, nasal congestion, nocturia, osteoarticular pain, polyuria, sexual difficulties.

The following postmarketing events have been reported infrequently in patients receiving CARDIZEM: alopecia, gingival hyperplasia, erythema multiforme, and leukopenia. However, a definitive cause and effect between these events and CARDIZEM therapy is yet to be established.

OVERDOSAGE OR EXAGGERATED RESPONSE

Overdosage experience with oral diltiazem has been limited. Single oral doses of 300 mg of CARDIZEM have been well tolerated by healthy volunteers. In the event of overdosage or exaggerated response, appropriate supportive measures should be employed in addition to gastric lavage. The following measures may be considered:

Bradycardia Administer atropine (0.60 to 1.0 mg). If there is no response to vagal blockade, administer isoproterenol cautiously.

High-Degree AV Block Treat as for bradycardia above. Fixed high-degree AV block should be treated with cardiac pacing.

Cardiac Failure Administer inotropic agents (isoproterenol, dopamine, or dobutamine) and diuretics.

Hypotension Vasopressors (eg, dopamine or levarterenol bitartrate).

Actual treatment and dosage should depend on the severity of the clinical situation and the judgment and experience of the treating physician.

The oral LD_{50}'s in mice and rats range from 415 to 740 mg/kg and from 560 to 810 mg/kg, respectively. The intravenous LD_{50}'s in these species were 60 and 38 mg/kg, respectively. The oral LD_{50} in dogs is considered to be in excess of 50 mg/kg, while lethality was seen in monkeys at 360 mg/kg. The toxic dose in man is not known. Due to extensive metabolism, blood levels after a standard dose of diltiazem can vary over tenfold, limiting the usefulness of blood levels in overdose cases. Overdoses with as much as 10.8 gm of oral diltiazem have been survived following appropriate supportive care.

DOSAGE AND ADMINISTRATION

Exertional Angina Pectoris Due to Atherosclerotic Coronary Artery Disease or Angina Pectoris at Rest Due to Coronary Artery Spasm. Dosage must be adjusted to each patient's needs. Starting with 30 mg four times daily, before meals and at bedtime, dosage should be increased gradually (given in divided doses three or four times daily) at one- to two-day intervals until optimum response is obtained. Although individual patients may respond to any dosage level, the average optimum dosage range appears to be 180 to 360 mg/day. There are no available data concerning dosage requirements in patients with impaired renal or hepatic function. If the drug must be used in such patients, titration should be carried out with particular caution.

Concomitant Use With Other Cardiovascular Agents.

1. **Sublingual NTG** may be taken as required to abort acute anginal attacks during CARDIZEM (diltiazem hydrochloride) therapy.

2. **Prophylactic Nitrate Therapy**—CARDIZEM may be safely coadminstered with short- and long-acting nitrates, but there have been no controlled studies to evaluate the antianginal effectiveness of this combination.

3. **Beta-blockers.** (See WARNINGS and PRECAUTIONS.)

HOW SUPPLIED

CARDIZEM 30-mg tablets are supplied in bottles of 100 (NDC 0088-1771-47) and 500 (NDC 0088-1771-55), and in Unit Dose Identification Paks of 100 (NDC 0088-1771-49). Each green tablet is engraved with MARION on one side and 1771 engraved on the other.

CARDIZEM 60-mg scored tablets are supplied in bottles of 90 (NDC 0088-1772-42), 100 (NDC 0088-1772-47), and 500 (NDC 0088-1772-55), and in Unit Dose Identification Paks of 100 (NDC 0088-1772-49). Each yellow tablet is engraved with MARION on one side and 1772 engraved on the other.

CARDIZEM 90-mg scored tablets are supplied in bottles of 90 (NDC 0088-1791-42), and 100 (NDC 0088-1791-47), and in Unit Dose Identification Paks of 100 (NDC 0088-1791-49). Each green oblong tablet is engraved with CARDIZEM on one side and 90 mg engraved on the other.

CARDIZEM 120-mg scored tablets are supplied in bottles of 90 (NDC 0088-1792-42), and 100 (NDC 0088-1792-47), and in Unit Dose Identification Paks of 100 (NDC 0088-1792-49). Each yellow oblong tablet is engraved with CARDIZEM on one side and 120 mg engraved on the other.

Store at controlled room temperature 59-86°F (15-30°C).

Issued 11/89

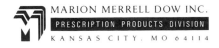
MARION MERRELL DOW INC.
PRESCRIPTION PRODUCTS DIVISION
KANSAS CITY, MO 64114

Professional Use Information

CARDIZEM® SR

(diltiazem hydrochloride)

Sustained Release Capsules

DESCRIPTION

CARDIZEM® (diltiazem hydrochloride) is a calcium ion influx inhibitor (slow channel blocker or calcium antagonist). Chemically, diltiazem hydrochloride is 1,5-Benzothiazepin-4(5H)one,3-(acetyloxy)-5-[2-(dimethylamino)ethyl]-2,3-dihydro-2-(4-methoxyphenyl)-, monohydrochloride, (+) -cis-. The chemical structure is:

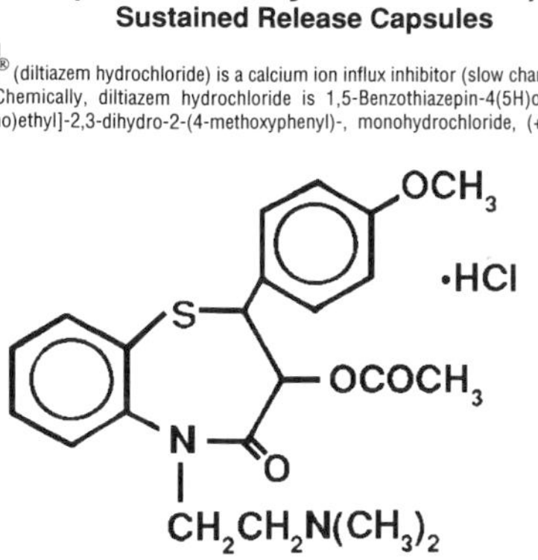

Diltiazem hydrochloride is a white to off-white crystalline powder with a bitter taste. It is soluble in water, methanol, and chloroform. It has a molecular weight of 450.98. Each CARDIZEM SR capsule contains either 60 mg, 90 mg, or 120 mg diltiazem hydrochloride.

Also contains: fumaric acid, povidone, starch, sucrose, talc, and other ingredients.

For oral administration.

CLINICAL PHARMACOLOGY

The therapeutic effects of CARDIZEM are believed to be related to its ability to inhibit the influx of calcium ions during membrane depolarization of cardiac and vascular smooth muscle.

Mechanisms of Action. CARDIZEM SR produces its antihypertensive effect primarily by relaxation of vascular smooth muscle and the resultant decrease in peripheral vascular resistance. The magnitude of blood pressure reduction is related to the degree of hypertension; thus hypertensive individuals experience an antihypertensive effect, whereas there is only a modest fall in blood pressure in normotensives.

Hemodynamic and Electrophysiologic Effects. Like other calcium antagonists, diltiazem decreases sinoatrial and atrioventricular conduction in isolated tissues and has a negative inotropic effect in isolated preparations. In the intact animal, prolongation of the AH interval can be seen at higher doses.

In man, diltiazem prevents spontaneous and ergonovine-provoked coronary artery spasm. It causes a decrease in peripheral vascular resistance and a modest fall in blood pressure in normotensive individuals and, in exercise tolerance studies in patients with ischemic heart disease, reduces the heart rate-blood pressure product for any given work load. Studies to date, primarily in patients with good ventricular function, have not revealed evidence of a negative inotropic effect; cardiac output, ejection fraction, and left ventricular end diastolic pressure have not been affected. Increased heart failure has, however, been reported in occasional patients with preexisting impairment of ventricular function. There are as yet few data on the interaction of diltiazem and beta-blockers in patients with poor ventricular function. Resting heart rate is usually slightly reduced by diltiazem.

CARDIZEM SR produces antihypertensive effects both in the supine and standing positions. Postural hypotension is infrequently noted upon suddenly assuming an upright position. No reflex tachycardia is associated with the chronic antihypertensive effects. CARDIZEM SR decreases vascular resistance, increases cardiac output (by increasing stroke volume), and produces a slight decrease or no change in heart rate. During dynamic exercise, increases in diastolic pressure are inhibited while maximum achievable systolic pressure is usually reduced. Heart rate at maximum exercise does not change or is slightly reduced. Chronic therapy with CARDIZEM produces no change or an increase in plasma catecholamines. No increased activity of the renin-angiotensin-aldosterone axis has been observed. CARDIZEM SR antagonizes the renal and peripheral effects of angiotensin II. Hypertensive animal models respond to diltiazem with reductions in blood pressure and increased urinary output and natriuresis without a change in urinary sodium/potassium ratio.

Intravenous diltiazem in doses of 20 mg prolongs AH conduction time and AV node functional and effective refractory periods approximately 20%. In a study involving single oral doses of 300 mg of CARDIZEM in six normal volunteers, the average maximum PR prolongation was 14% with no instances of greater than first-degree AV block. Diltiazem-associated prolongation of the AH interval is not more pronounced in patients with first-degree heart block. In patients with sick sinus syndrome, diltiazem significantly prolongs sinus cycle length (up to 50% in some cases).

Chronic oral administration of CARDIZEM in doses of up to 360 mg/day has resulted in small increases in PR interval, and on occasion produces abnormal prolongation. (See WARNINGS.)

Pharmacokinetics and Metabolism. Diltiazem is well absorbed from the gastrointestinal tract and is subject to an extensive first-pass effect, giving an absolute bioavailability (compared to intravenous administration) of about 40%. CARDIZEM undergoes extensive metabolism in which 2% to 4% of the unchanged drug appears in the urine. In vitro binding studies show CARDIZEM is 70% to 80% bound to plasma proteins. Competitive in vitro ligand binding studies have also shown CARDIZEM binding is not altered by therapeutic concentrations of digoxin, hydrochlorothiazide, phenylbutazone, propranolol, salicylic acid, or warfarin. The plasma elimination half-life following single or multiple drug administration is approximately 3.0 to 4.5 hours. Desacetyl diltiazem is also present in the plasma at levels of 10% to 20% of the parent drug and is 25% to 50% as potent a coronary vasodilator as diltiazem. Minimum therapeutic plasma levels of CARDIZEM appear to be in the range of 50-200 ng/mL. There is a departure from linearity when dose strengths are increased; the half-life is slightly increased with dose. A study that compared patients with normal hepatic function to patients with cirrhosis found an increase in half-life and a 69% increase in bioavailability in the hepatically impaired patients. A single study in patients with severely impaired renal function showed no difference in the pharmacokinetic profile of diltiazem compared to patients with normal renal function.

Cardizem SR Capsules. Diltiazem is absorbed from the capsule formulation to about 92% of a reference solution at steady-state. A single 120-mg dose of the capsule results in detectable plasma levels within two to three hours and peak plasma levels at six to 11 hours. The apparent elimination half-life after single or multiple dosing is five to seven hours. A departure from linearity similar to that observed with the CARDIZEM tablet is observed. As the dose of CARDIZEM SR capsules is increased from a daily dose of 120 mg (60 mg bid) to 240 mg (120 mg bid) daily, there is an increase in bioavailability of 2.6 times. When the dose is increased from 240 mg to 360 mg daily there is an increase in bioavailability of 1.8 times. The average plasma levels of the capsule dosed twice daily at steady-state are equivalent to the tablet dosed four times daily when the same total daily dose is administered.

INDICATIONS AND USAGE

CARDIZEM SR is indicated for the treatment of hypertension. It may be used alone or in combination with other antihypertensive medications, such as diuretics.

CONTRAINDICATIONS

CARDIZEM is contraindicated in (1) patients with sick sinus syndrome except in the presence of a functioning ventricular pacemaker, (2) patients with second- or third-degree AV block except in the presence of a functioning ventricular pacemaker, (3) patients with hypotension (less than 90 mm Hg systolic), (4) patients who have demonstrated hypersensitivity to the drug, and (5) patients with acute myocardial infarction and pulmonary congestion documented by x-ray on admission.

WARNINGS

1. Cardiac Conduction. CARDIZEM prolongs AV node refractory periods without significantly prolonging sinus node recovery time, except in patients with sick sinus syndrome. This effect may rarely result in abnormally slow heart rates (particularly in patients with sick sinus syndrome) or second- or third-degree AV block (nine of 2,111 patients or 0.43%). Concomitant use of diltiazem with beta-blockers or digitalis may result in additive effects on cardiac conduction. A patient with Prinzmetal's angina developed periods of asystole (2 to 5 seconds) after a single dose of 60 mg of diltiazem.

2. Congestive Heart Failure. Although diltiazem has a negative inotropic effect in isolated animal tissue preparations, hemodynamic studies in humans with normal ventricular function have not shown a reduction in cardiac index nor consistent negative effects on contractility (dp/dt). An acute study of oral diltiazem in patients with impaired ventricular function (ejection fraction 24% ± 6%) showed improvement in indices of ventricular function without significant decrease in contractile function (dp/dt). Experience with the use of CARDIZEM (diltiazem hydrochloride) in combination with beta-blockers in patients with impaired ventricular function is limited. Caution should be exercised when using this combination.

3. Hypotension. Decreases in blood pressure associated with CARDIZEM therapy may occasionally result in symptomatic hypotension.

4. Acute Hepatic Injury. Mild elevations of transaminases with and without concomitant elevation in alkaline phosphatase and bilirubin have been observed in clinical studies. Such elevations were usually transient and frequently resolved even with continued diltiazem treatment. In rare instances, significant elevations in enzymes such as alkaline phosphatase, LDH, SGOT, SGPT, and other phenomena consistent with acute hepatic injury have been noted. These reactions tended to occur early after therapy initiation (1 to 8 weeks) and have been reversible upon discontinuation of drug therapy. The relationship to CARDIZEM is uncertain in some cases , but probable in some. (See PRECAUTIONS.)

PRECAUTIONS

General. CARDIZEM (diltiazem hydrochloride) is extensively metabolized by the liver and excreted by the kidneys and in bile. As with any drug given over prolonged periods, laboratory parameters should be monitored at regular intervals. The drug should be used with caution in patients with impaired renal or hepatic function. In subacute and chronic dog and rat studies designed to produce toxicity, high doses of diltiazem were associated with hepatic damage. In special subacute hepatic studies, oral doses of 125 mg/kg and higher in rats were associated with histological changes in the liver which were reversible when the drug was discontinued. In dogs, doses of 20 mg/kg were also associated with hepatic changes; however, these changes were reversible with continued dosing.

Dermatological events (see ADVERSE REACTIONS section) may be transient and may disappear despite continued use of CARDIZEM. However, skin eruptions progressing to erythema multiforme and/or exfoliative dermatitis have also been infrequently reported. Should a dermatologic reaction persist, the drug should be discontinued.

Drug Interaction. Due to the potential for additive effects, caution and careful titration are warranted in patients receiving CARDIZEM concomitantly with any agents known to affect cardiac contractility and/or conduction. (See WARNINGS.) Pharmacologic studies indicate that there may be additive effects in prolonging AV conduction when using beta-blockers or digitalis concomitantly with CARDIZEM. (See WARNINGS.)

As with all drugs, care should be exercised when treating patients with multiple medications. CARDIZEM undergoes biotransformation by cytochrome P-450 mixed function oxidase. Coadministration of CARDIZEM with other agents which follow the same route of biotransformation may result in the competitive inhibition of metabolism. Dosages of similarly metabolized drugs, particularly those of low therapeutic ratio or in patients with renal and/or hepatic impairment, may require adjustment when starting or stopping concomitantly administered CARDIZEM to maintain optimum therapeutic blood levels.

Beta-blockers: Controlled and uncontrolled domestic studies suggest that concomitant use of CARDIZEM and beta-blockers or digitalis is usually well tolerated, but available data are not sufficient to predict the effects of concomitant treatment in patients with left ventricular dysfunction or cardiac conduction abnormalities.

Administration of CARDIZEM (diltiazem hydrochloride) concomitantly with propranolol in five normal volunteers resulted in increased propranolol levels in all subjects and bio-availability of propranolol was increased approximately 50%. If combination therapy is initiated or withdrawn in conjunction with propranolol, an adjustment in the propranolol dose may be warranted. (See WARNINGS.)

Cimetidine: A study in six healthy volunteers has shown a significant increase in peak diltiazem plasma levels (58%) and area-under-the-curve (53%) after a 1-week course of cimetidine at 1,200 mg per day and diltiazem 60 mg per day. Ranitidine produced smaller, nonsignificant increases. The effect may be mediated by cimetidine's known inhibition of hepatic cytochrome P-450, the enzyme system probably responsible for the first-pass metabolism of diltiazem. Patients currently receiving diltiazem therapy should be carefully monitored for a change in pharmacological effect when initiating and discontinuing therapy with cimetidine. An adjustment in the diltiazem dose may be warranted.

Digitalis: Administration of CARDIZEM with digoxin in 24 healthy male subjects increased plasma digoxin concentrations approximately 20%. Another investigator found no increase in digoxin levels in 12 patients with coronary artery disease. Since there have been conflicting results regarding the effect of digoxin levels, it is recommended that digoxin levels be monitored when initiating, adjusting, and discontinuing CARDIZEM therapy to avoid possible over- or under-digitalization. (See WARNINGS.)

Anesthetics: The depression of cardiac contractility, conductivity, and automaticity as well as the vascular dilation associated with anesthetics may be potentiated by calcium channel blockers. When used concomitantly, anesthetics and calcium blockers should be titrated carefully.

Carcinogenesis, Mutagenesis, Impairment of Fertility. A 24-month study in rats and a 21-month study in mice showed no evidence of carcinogenicity. There was also no mutagenic response in in vitro bacterial tests. No intrinsic effect on fertility was observed in rats.

Pregnancy. Category C. Reproduction studies have been conducted in mice, rats, and rabbits. Administration of doses ranging from five to ten times greater (on a mg/kg basis) than the daily recommended therapeutic dose has resulted in embryo and fetal lethality. These doses, in some studies, have been reported to cause skeletal abnormalities. In the perinatal/postnatal studies, there was some reduction in early individual pup weights and survival rates. There was an increased incidence of stillbirths at doses of 20 times the human dose or greater.

CARDIZEM® SR
(diltiazem hydrochloride)
Sustained Release Capsules

There are no well-controlled studies in pregnant women; therefore, use CARDIZEM in pregnant women only if the potential benefit justifies the potential risk to the fetus.

Nursing Mothers. Diltiazem is excreted in human milk. One report suggests that concentrations in breast milk may approximate serum levels. If use of CARDIZEM is deemed essential, an alternative method of infant feeding should be instituted.

Pediatric Use. Safety and effectiveness in children have not been established.

ADVERSE REACTIONS

Serious adverse reactions have been rare in studies carried out to date, but it should be recognized that patients with impaired ventricular function and cardiac conduction abnormalities have usually been excluded from these studies.

The adverse events described below represent events observed in clinical studies of hypertensive patients receiving either CARDIZEM Tablets or CARDIZEM SR Capsules as well as experiences observed in studies of angina and during marketing. The most common events in hypertension studies are shown in a table with rates in placebo patients shown for comparison. Less common events are listed by body system; these include any adverse reactions seen in angina studies that were not observed in hypertension studies. In all hypertensive patients studied (over 900), the most common adverse events were edema (9%), headache (8%), dizziness (6%), asthenia (5%), sinus bradycardia (3%), flushing (3%), and 1° AV block (3%). Only edema and perhaps bradycardia and dizziness were dose related. The most common events observed in clinical studies (over 2,100 patients) of angina patients and hypertensive patients receiving CARDIZEM Tablets or CARDIZEM SR Capsules were (ie, greater than 1%) edema (5.4%), headache (4.5%), dizziness (3.4%), asthenia (2.8%), first-degree AV block (1.8%), flushing (1.7%), nausea (1.6%), bradycardia (1.5%), and rash (1.5%).

DOUBLE BLIND PLACEBO CONTROLLED HYPERTENSION TRIALS		
Adverse	**Diltiazem** N=315 # pts (%)	**Placebo** N=211 # pts (%)
headache	38 (12%)	17 (8%)
AV block first degree	24 (7.6%)	4 (1.9%)
dizziness	22 (7%)	6 (2.8%)
edema	19 (6%)	2 (0.9%)
bradycardia	19 (6%)	3 (1.4%)
ECG abnormality	13 (4.1%)	3 (1.4%)
asthenia	10 (3.2%)	1 (0.5%)
constipation	5 (1.6%)	2 (0.9%)
dyspepsia	4 (1.3%)	1 (0.5%)
nausea	4 (1.3%)	2 (0.9%)
palpitations	4 (1.3%)	2 (0.9%)
polyuria	4 (1.3%)	2 (0.9%)
somnolence	4 (1.3%)	—
alk phos increase	3 (1%)	1 (0.5%)
hypotension	3 (1%)	1 (0.5%)
insomnia	3 (1%)	1 (0.5%)
rash	3 (1%)	1 (0.5%)
AV block second degree	2 (0.6%)	—

In addition, the following events were reported infrequently (less than 1%) or have been observed in angina trials. In many cases, the relation to drug is uncertain.

Cardiovascular: Angina, arrhythmia, bundle branch block, tachycardia, ventricular extrasystoles, congestive heart failure, syncope.

Nervous System: Amnesia, depression, gait abnormality, hallucinations, nervousness, paresthesia, personality change, tinnitus, tremor, abnormal dreams.

Gastrointestinal: Anorexia, diarrhea, dysgeusia, mild elevations of SGOT, SGPT, and LDH (see hepatic warnings), vomiting, weight increase, thirst.

Dermatological: Petechiae, pruritus, photosensitivity, urticaria.

Other: Amblyopia, CPK increase, dyspnea, epistaxis, eye irritation, hyperglycemia, sexual difficulties, nasal congestion, nocturia, osteoarticular pain, impotence, dry mouth.

The following postmarketing events have been reported infrequently in patients receiving CARDIZEM: alopecia, gingival hyperplasia, erythema multiforme, and leukopenia. Definitive cause and effect relationship between these events and CARDIZEM therapy cannot yet be established.

OVERDOSAGE OR EXAGGERATED RESPONSE

Overdosage experience with oral diltiazem has been limited. Single oral doses of 300 mg of CARDIZEM have been well tolerated by healthy volunteers. In the event of overdosage or exaggerated response, appropriate supportive measures should be employed in addition to gastric lavage. The following measures may be considered:

Bradycardia: Administer atropine (0.60 to 1.0 mg). If there is no response to vagal blockade, administer isoproterenol cautiously.

High-Degree AV Block: Treat as for bradycardia above. Fixed high-degree AV blockshould be treated with cardiac pacing.

Cardiac Failure: Administer inotropic agents (isoproterenol, dopamine, or dobutamine) and diuretics.

Hypotension: Vasopressors (eg, dopamine or levarterenol bitartrate).

Actual treatment and dosage should depend on the severity of the clinical situation and the judgment and experience of the treating physician.

The oral LD_{50}'s in mice and rats range from 415 to 740 mg/kg and from 560 to 810 mg/kg, respectively. The intravenous LD_{50}'s in these species were 60 and 38 mg/kg, respectively. The oral LD_{50} in dogs is considered to be in excess of 50 mg/kg, while lethality was seen in monkeys at 360 mg/kg. The toxic dose in man is not known. Due to extensive metabolism, blood levels after a standard dose of diltiazem can vary over tenfold, limiting the usefulness of blood levels in overdose cases. Overdoses with as much as 10.8 gm of oral diltiazem have been survived following appropriate supportive care.

DOSAGE AND ADMINISTRATION

Dosages must be adjusted to each patient's needs, starting with 60 to 120 mg twice daily. Maximum antihypertensive effect is usually observed by 14 days of chronic therapy; therefore, dosage adjustments should be scheduled accordingly. Although individual patients may respond to lower doses, the usual optimum dosage range in clinical trials was 240 to 360 mg/day.

CARDIZEM SR has an additive antihypertensive effect when used with other antihypertensive agents. Therefore, the dosage of CARDIZEM SR or the concomitant antihypertensives may need to be adjusted when adding one to the other. See WARNINGS and PRECAUTIONS regarding use with beta-blockers.

HOW SUPPLIED

CARDIZEM® SR (diltiazem hydrochloride) Sustained Release Capsules			
Strength	Quantity	NDC Number	Description
60 mg	100 btl 100 UDIP®	0088-1777-47 0088-1777-49	Ivory/brown capsule imprinted with CARDIZEM logo on one end and CARDIZEM SR 60 mg on the other
90 mg	100 btl 100 UDIP®	0088-1778-47 0088-1778-49	Gold/brown capsule imprinted with CARDIZEM logo on one end and CARDIZEM SR 90 mg on the other
120 mg	100 btl 100 UDIP®	0088-1779-47 0088-1779-49	Caramel/brown capsule imprinted with CARDIZEM logo on one end and CARDIZEM SR 120 mg on the other

Storage Conditions: Store at controlled room temperature 59-86°F (15-30°C).

Issued 1/89

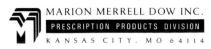

MARION MERRELL DOW INC.
PRESCRIPTION PRODUCTS DIVISION
KANSAS CITY, MO 64114

Seldane®
(terfenadine) 60 mg Tablets

CAUTION: Federal law prohibits dispensing without prescription.

DESCRIPTION

Seldane (terfenadine) is available as tablets for oral administration. Each tablet contains 60 mg terfenadine. Tablets also contain, as inactive ingredients: corn starch, gelatin, lactose, magnesium stearate, and sodium bicarbonate.

Terfenadine is a histamine H_1-receptor antagonist with the chemical name α-[4-(1,1-Dimethylethyl) phenyl]-4-(hydroxydiphenylmethyl)-1-piperidinebutanol ($\pm$). The molecular weight is 471.68. The molecular formula is $C_{32}H_{41}NO_2$.

It has the following chemical structure:

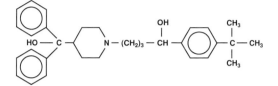

Terfenadine occurs as a white to off-white crystalline powder. It is freely soluble in chloroform, soluble in ethanol, and very slightly soluble in water.

CLINICAL PHARMACOLOGY

Terfenadine is chemically and pharmacologically distinct from other antihistamines.

Histamine skin wheal studies have shown that Seldane in single and repeated doses of 60 mg in 64 subjects has an antihistaminic effect beginning at 1-2 hours, reaching its maximum at 3-4 hours, and lasting in excess of 12 hours.

Clinical trials of Seldane involved about 2,600 patients, most receiving either Seldane, another antihistamine and/or placebo in double-blind, randomized controlled comparisons. The four best controlled and largest trials each lasted 7 days and involved about 1,000 total patients in comparisons of Seldane (60 mg b.i.d.) with an active drug (chlorpheniramine, 4 mg t.i.d.; dexchlorpheniramine, 2 mg t.i.d.; or clemastine 1 mg b.i.d.). In the four trials, about 50-70% of Seldane or other antihistamine recipients had moderate to complete relief of symptoms, compared with 30-50% of placebo recipients, with a significant difference favoring the active drugs in each study. In these studies, Seldane was associated with less frequent drowsiness than the other antihistamines; the frequency of drowsiness with Seldane was similar to the frequency with placebo. None of these studies showed a difference between Seldane and other antihistamines in the frequency of anticholinergic effects. In studies which included 52 subjects in whom EEG assessments were made, no depressant effects have been observed.

Animal studies have demonstrated that terfenadine is a histamine H_1-receptor antagonist. In these animal studies, no sedative or anticholinergic effects were observed at effective antihistaminic doses. Radioactive disposition and autoradiographic studies in rats and radioligand binding studies with guinea pig brain H_1-receptors indicate that, at effective antihistamine doses, neither terfenadine nor its metabolites penetrate the blood brain barrier well.

Relative to a terfenadine suspension, terfenadine tablets are equally bioavailable. On the basis of a mass balance study using ¹⁴C labelled terfenadine the oral absorption of terfenadine was estimated to be at least 70%. Terfenadine itself undergoes extensive (99%) first pass metabolism to two primary metabolites, an active acid metabolite and an inactive dealkylated metabolite. Therefore, systemic availability of terfenadine would be low. From information gained in the ¹⁴C study it appears that approximately forty percent of the total dose is eliminated renally (40% of this as acid metabolite, 30% dealkyl metabolite, and 30% minor unidentified metabolites). Sixty percent of the dose is eliminated in the feces (50% of it as the acid metabolite, 2% unchanged terfenadine, and the remainder as minor unidentified metabolites). Studies investigating the effect of hepatic and renal insufficiency on the metabolism and excretion of terfenadine are incomplete. Preliminary information indicates that in cases of hepatic impairment, significant concentrations of unchanged terfenadine can be detected with the rate of acid metabolite formation being decreased. In subjects with normal hepatic function unchanged terfenadine plasma concentrations have not been detected.

In vitro studies demonstrate that terfenadine is extensively (97%) bound to human serum protein while the acid metabolite is approximately 70% bound to human serum protein. Based on data gathered from in vitro models of antihistaminic activity, the acid metabolite of terfenadine has approximately 30% of the H_1 blocking activity of terfenadine. The relative contribution of terfenadine and the acid metabolite to the pharmacodynamic effects have not been clearly defined. Since unchanged terfenadine is usually not detected in plasma and active acid metabolite concentrations are relatively high, the acid metabolite may be the entity responsible for the majority of efficacy after oral administration of terfenadine.

In a study involving the administration of a single 60 mg Seldane tablet to 24 subjects, mean peak plasma levels of the acid metabolite were 263 ng/mL (range 133-423 ng/mL) and occurred approximately 2.5 hours after dosing. Plasma concentrations of unchanged terfenadine were not detected. The elimination profile of the acid metabolite was biphasic in nature with an initial mean plasma half-life of 3.5 hours followed by a mean plasma half-life of 6 hours. Ninety percent of the plasma level time curve was associated with these half-lives. Preliminary evidence exists at doses four times of that currently approved, that there may emerge a third phase with a half-life of >14 hours. This third phase was associated with about twenty percent of the plasma level time curve.

After multiple dose administration to steady-state of 60 mg Seldane tablets every 12 hours the observed accumulation of Area Under the Curve during the dosing interval for the active acid metabolite was 1.6[1]. This observed accumulation factor corresponds to an effective pharmacokinetic half-life of 8.5 hours. This 8.5 hour half-life would predict time to steady-state, steady-state concentrations as well as time for drug elimination after multiple dosing.

[1]Observed Accumulation Factor= ᴬᵁᶜ0-12 at steady-state/ᴬᵁᶜ0-12 first dose

INDICATIONS AND USAGE

Seldane is indicated for the relief of symptoms associated with seasonal allergic rhinitis such as sneezing, rhinorrhea, pruritus, and lacrimation.

CONTRAINDICATIONS

Seldane is contraindicated in patients with a known hypersensitivity to terfenadine or any of its ingredients.

PRECAUTIONS

General

Terfenadine undergoes extensive metabolism in the liver. Patients with impaired hepatic function (alcoholic cirrhosis, hepatitis), or on ketoconazole or troleandomycin therapy, or having conditions leading to QT prolongation (e.g., hypokalemia, congenital QT syndrome) may experience QT prolongation and/or ventricular tachycardia at the recommended dose. The effect of terfenadine in patients who are receiving agents which alter the QT interval is not known. These events have also occurred in patients on macrolide antibiotics, including erythromycin, but causality is unclear. The events may be related to altered metabolism of the drug, to electrolyte imbalance, or both.

Information for Patients

Patients taking Seldane should receive the following information and instructions. Antihistamines are prescribed to reduce allergic symptoms. Patients should be questioned about pregnancy or lactation before starting Seldane therapy, since the drug should be used in pregnancy or lactation only if the potential benefit justifies the potential risk to fetus or baby. Patients should be instructed to take Seldane only as needed and not to exceed the prescribed dose. Patients should also be instructed to store this medication in a tightly closed container in a cool, dry place, away from heat or direct sunlight, and away from children.

Drug Interactions

Preliminary evidence exists that concurrent ketoconazole or macrolide administration significantly alters the metabolism of terfenadine. Concurrent use of Seldane with ketoconazole or troleandomycin is not recommended. Concurrent use of other macrolides should be approached with caution.

Carcinogenesis, mutagenesis, impairment of fertility

Oral doses of terfenadine, corresponding to 63 times the recommended human daily dose, in mice for 18 months or in rats for 24 months, revealed no evidence of tumorigenicity. Microbial and micronucleus test assays with terfenadine have revealed no evidence of mutagenesis.

Reproduction and fertility studies in rats showed no effects on male or female fertility at oral doses of up to 21 times the human daily dose. At 63 times the human daily dose there was a small but significant reduction in implants and at 125 times the human daily dose reduced implants and increased post-implantation losses were observed, which were judged to be secondary to maternal toxicity.

Pregnancy Category C

There was no evidence of animal teratogenicity. Reproduction studies have been performed in rats at doses 63 times and 125 times the human daily dose and have revealed decreased pup weight gain and survival when terfenadine was administered throughout pregnancy and lactation. There are no adequate and well-controlled studies in pregnant women. Seldane should be used during pregnancy only if the potential benefit justifies the potential risk to the fetus.

Nonteratogenic effects

Seldane is not recommended for nursing women. The drug has caused decreased pup weight gain and survival in rats given doses 63 times and 125 times the human daily dose throughout pregnancy and lactation. Effects on pups exposed to Seldane only during lactation are not known, and there are no adequate and well-controlled studies in women during lactation.

Pediatric use

Safety and effectiveness of Seldane in children below the age of 12 years have not been established.

ADVERSE REACTIONS

Experience from clinical studies, including both controlled and uncontrolled studies involving more than 2,400 patients who received Seldane, provides information on adverse experience incidence for periods of a few days up to six months. The usual dose in these studies was 60 mg twice daily, but in a small number of patients, the dose was as low as 20 mg twice a day, or as high as 600 mg daily.

In controlled clinical studies using the recommended dose of 60 mg b.i.d., the incidence of reported adverse effects in patients receiving Seldane was similar to that reported in patients receiving placebo. (See Table below.)

ADVERSE EVENTS REPORTED IN CLINICAL TRIALS

	Percent of Patients Reporting				
	Controlled Studies*			All Clinical Studies**	
Adverse Event	Seldane N=781	Placebo N=665	Control N=626***	Seldane N=2462	Placebo N=1478
Central Nervous System					
Drowsiness	9.0	8.1	18.1	8.5	8.2
Headache	6.3	7.4	3.8	15.8	11.2
Fatigue	2.9	0.9	5.8	4.5	3.0
Dizziness	1.4	1.1	1.0	1.5	1.2
Nervousness	0.9	0.2	0.5	1.7	1.0
Weakness	0.9	0.6	0.2	0.6	0.5
Appetite Increase	0.6	0.0	0.0	0.5	0.0
Gastrointestinal System					
Gastrointestinal Distress (Abdominal Distress, Nausea, Vomiting, Change in Bowel Habits)	4.6	3.0	2.7	7.6	5.4
Eye, Ear, Nose, and Throat					
Dry Mouth/Nose/Throat	2.3	1.8	3.5	4.8	3.1
Cough	0.9	0.2	0.5	2.5	1.7
Sore Throat	0.5	0.3	0.5	3.2	1.6
Epistaxis	0.0	0.8	0.2	0.7	0.4
Skin					
Eruption (including rash and urticaria) or Itching	1.0	1.7	1.4	1.6	2.0

* Duration of treatment in "CONTROLLED STUDIES" was usually 7-14 days.
** Duration of treatment in "ALL CLINICAL STUDIES" was up to 6 months.
*** CONTROL DRUGS: Chlorpheniramine (291 patients), d-Chlorpheniramine (189 patients), Clemastine (146 patients)

Seldane®
(terfenadine) 60 mg Tablets

Rare reports of severe cardiovascular adverse effects have been received which include arrhythmias (ventricular tachyarrhythmia, torsades de pointes, ventricular fibrillation), hypotension, palpitations, and syncope. In controlled clinical trials in otherwise normal patients with rhinitis, at doses of 60 mg b.i.d. small increases in QTc interval were observed. Changes of this magnitude in a normal population are of doubtful clinical significance. However, in another study (N=20 patients) at 300 mg b.i.d. a mean increase in QTc of 10% (range -4% to +30%)(mean increase of 46 msec) was observed without clinical sign or symptoms.

In addition to the more frequent side effects reported in clinical trials (See Table), adverse effects have been reported at a lower incidence in clinical trials and/or spontaneously during marketing of Seldane that warrant listing as possibly associated with drug administration. These include: alopecia (hair loss or thinning), anaphylaxis, angioedema, bronchospasm, confusion, depression, galactorrhea, insomnia, menstrual disorders (including dysmenorrhea), musculoskeletal symptoms, nightmares, paresthesia, photosensitivity, seizures, sinus tachycardia, sweating, tremor, urinary frequency, and visual disturbances.

In clinical trials, several instances of mild, or in one case, moderate transaminase elevations were seen in patients receiving Seldane. Mild elevations were also seen in placebo treated patients. Marketing experiences include isolated reports of jaundice, cholestatic hepatitis, and hepatitis. In most cases available information is incomplete.

OVERDOSAGE

Generally, signs and symptoms of overdosage are absent or mild (e.g., headache, nausea, confusion). At overdoses of 600 mg/day (300 mg b.i.d.) there may be prolongation of the QT interval. At 900 mg or more there have been rare incidents of ventricular arrhythmia (torsades de pointes or fibrillation). Seizures and syncope have been reported.

Therefore, in cases of overdosage, cardiac monitoring for at least 24 hours is recommended and for as long as QTc is prolonged, along with standard measures to remove any unabsorbed drug. Limited experience with the use of hemoperfusion (N=1) or hemodialysis (N=3) was not successful in completely removing the acid metabolite of terfenadine from the blood.

Treatment of the signs and symptoms of overdosage should be symptomatic and supportive after the acute stage.

Oral LD_{50} values for terfenadine were greater than 5000 mg/kg in mature mice and rats. The oral LD_{50} was 438 mg/kg in newborn rats.

DOSAGE AND ADMINISTRATION

One tablet (60 mg) twice daily for adults and children 12 years and older.

HOW SUPPLIED

NDC 0068-0723-61
   60 mg tablets in bottles of 100.
NDC 0068-0723-65
   60 mg tablets in bottles of 500.
   Tablets are round, white, and debossed "SELDANE". Store tablets at controlled room temperature (59°-86°F) (15°-30°C). Protect from exposure to temperatures above 104°F (40°C) and moisture.
   Product Information as of July, 1990

J173H

U.S. Patent 3,878,217
Other patent applications pending.

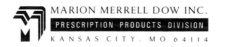

MARION MERRELL DOW INC.
PRESCRIPTION PRODUCTS DIVISION
KANSAS CITY, MO 64114

CARAFATE® Tablets
(sucralfate)

DESCRIPTION

CARAFATE® (sucralfate) is α-D-Glucopyranoside, β-D-fructofuranosyl-, octakis-(hydrogen sulfate), aluminum complex.

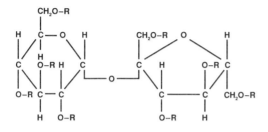

$$R = SO_3[Al_2(OH)_5 \cdot (H_2O)_2]$$

Tablets for oral administration contain 1 gm of sucralfate.

Also contain: D&C Red #30 Lake, FD&C Blue #1 Lake, magnesium stearate, microcrystalline cellulose, and starch.

Therapeutic category: antiulcer

CLINICAL PHARMACOLOGY

Sucralfate is only minimally absorbed from the gastrointestinal tract. The small amounts of the sulfated disaccharide that are absorbed are excreted primarily in the urine.

Although the mechanism of sucralfate's ability to accelerate healing of duodenal ulcers remains to be fully defined, it is known that it exerts its effect through a local, rather than systemic, action. The following observations also appear pertinent:

1. Studies in human subjects and with animal models of ulcer disease have shown that sucralfate forms an ulcer-adherent complex with proteinaceous exudate at the ulcer site.

2. In vitro, a sucralfate-albumin film provides a barrier to diffusion of hydrogen ions.

3. In human subjects, sucralfate given in doses recommended for ulcer therapy inhibits pepsin activity in gastric juice by 32%.

4. In vitro, sucralfate adsorbs bile salts.

These observations suggest that sucralfate's antiulcer activity is the result of formation of an ulcer-adherent complex that covers the ulcer site and protects it against further attack by acid, pepsin, and bile salts. There are approximately 14-16 mEq of acid neutralizing capacity per 1-gm dose of sucralfate.

CLINICAL TRIALS

Acute Duodenal Ulcer

Over 600 patients have participated in well-controlled clinical trials worldwide. Multicenter trials conducted in the United States, both of them placebo-controlled studies with endoscopic evaluation at 2 and 4 weeks, showed:

STUDY 1

Treatment Groups	Ulcer Healing/No. Patients	
	2 wk	4 wk (Overall)
Sucralfate	37/105 (35.2%)	82/109 (75.2%)
Placebo	26/106 (24.5%)	68/107 (63.6%)

STUDY 2

Treatment Groups	Ulcer Healing/No. Patients	
	2 wk	4 wk (Overall)
Sucralfate	8/24 (33%)	22/24 (92%)
Placebo	4/31 (13%)	18/31 (58%)

The sucralfate-placebo differences were statistically significant in both studies at 4 weeks but not at 2 weeks. The poorer result in the first study may have occurred because sucralfate was given 2 hours after meals and at bedtime rather than 1 hour before meals and at bedtime, the regimen used in international studies and in the second United States study. In addition, in the first study liquid antacid was utilized as needed, whereas in the second study antacid tablets were used.

Maintenance Therapy After Healing of Duodenal Ulcer

Two double-blind randomized placebo-controlled U.S. multicenter trials have demonstrated that sucralfate (1 gm bid) is effective as maintenance therapy following healing of duodenal ulcers.

In one study, endoscopies were performed monthly for 4 months. Of the 254 patients who enrolled, 239 were analyzed in the intention-to-treat life table analysis presented below.

Duodenal Ulcer Recurrence Rate (%)					
		Months of Therapy			
Drug	N	1	2	3	4
Carafate	122	20*	30*	38**	42**
Placebo	117	33	46	55	63

*$p < 0.05$, **$p < 0.01$

PRN antacids were not permitted in this study.

In the other study, scheduled endoscopies were performed at 6 and 12 months, but for cause endoscopies were permitted as symptoms dictated. Median symptom scores between the sucralfate and placebo groups were not significantly different. A life table intention-to-treat analysis for the 94 patients enrolled in the trial had the following results:

Duodenal Ulcer Recurrence Rate (%)			
Drug	N	6 months	12 months
Carafate	48	19*	27*
Placebo	46	54	65

*$p < 0.002$

PRN antacids were permitted in this study.

Data from placebo-controlled studies longer than 1 year are not available.

INDICATIONS AND USAGE

CARAFATE® (sucralfate) is indicated in:

1. Short-term treatment (up to 8 weeks) of active duodenal ulcer. While healing with sucralfate may occur during the first week or two, treatment should be continued for 4 to 8 weeks unless healing has been demonstrated by x-ray or endoscopic examination.

2. Maintenance therapy for duodenal ulcer patients at reduced dosage after healing of acute ulcers.

CONTRAINDICATIONS

There are no known contraindications to the use of sucralfate.

PRECAUTIONS

Duodenal ulcer is a chronic, recurrent disease. While short term treatment with sucralfate can result in complete healing of the ulcer, a successful course of treatment with sucralfate should not be expected to alter the post-healing frequency or severity of duodenal ulceration.

Special Populations: Chronic Renal Failure and Dialysis Patients: When sucralfate is administered orally, small amounts of aluminum are absorbed from the gastrointestinal tract. Concomitant use of sucralfate with other products that contain aluminum, such as aluminum-containing antacids, may increase the total body burden of aluminum. Patients with normal renal function receiving the recommended doses of sucralfate and aluminum-containing products adequately excrete aluminum in the urine. Patients with chronic renal failure or those receiving dialysis have impaired excretion of absorbed aluminum. In addition, aluminum does not cross dialysis membranes because it is bound to albumin and transferrin plasma proteins. Aluminum accumulation and toxicity (aluminum osteodystrophy, osteomalacia, encephalopathy) have been described in patients with renal impairment. Sucralfate should be used with caution in patients with chronic renal failure.

Drug Interactions: Some studies have shown that simultaneous sucralfate administration in healthy volunteers reduced the extent of absorption (bioavailability) of single doses of the following drugs: cimetidine, ciprofloxacin, digoxin, norfloxacin, phenytoin, ranitidine, tetracycline, and theophylline. The mechanism of these interactions appears to be nonsystemic in nature, presumably resulting from sucralfate binding to the concomitant agent in the gastrointestinal tract. In all cases studied to date (cimetidine, ciprofloxacin, digoxin, and ranitidine), dosing the concomitant medication 2 hours before sucralfate eliminated the interaction. Because of the potential of CARAFATE to alter the absorption of some drugs, CARAFATE should be administered separately from other drugs when alterations in bioavailability are felt to be critical. In these cases, patients should be monitored appropriately.

Carcinogenesis, Mutagenesis, Impairment of Fertility: Chronic oral toxicity studies of 24 months' duration were conducted in mice and rats at doses up to 1 gm/kg (12 times the human dose). There was no evidence of drug-related tumorigenicity. A reproduction study in rats at doses up to 38 times the human dose did not reveal any indication of fertility impairment. Mutagenicity studies were not conducted.

Pregnancy: Teratogenic effects. Pregnancy Category B. Teratogenicity studies have been performed in mice, rats, and rabbits at doses up to 50 times the human dose and have revealed no evidence of harm to the fetus due to sucralfate. There are, however, no adequate and well-controlled studies in pregnant women. Because animal reproduction studies are not always predictive of human response, this drug should be used during pregnancy only if clearly needed.

CARAFATE® Tablets
(sucralfate)

Nursing Mothers: It is not known whether this drug is excreted in human milk. Because many drugs are excreted in human milk, caution should be exercised when sucralfate is administered to a nursing woman.

Pediatric Use: Safety and effectiveness in children have not been established.

ADVERSE REACTIONS

Adverse reactions to sucralfate in clinical trials were minor and only rarely led to discontinuation of the drug. In studies involving over 2700 patients treated with sucralfate tablets, adverse effects were reported in 129 (4.7%).

Constipation was the most frequent complaint (2%). Other adverse effects reported in less than 0.5% of the patients are listed below by body system:

Gastrointestinal: diarrhea, nausea, vomiting, gastric discomfort, indigestion, flatulence, dry mouth

Dermatological: pruritus, rash

Nervous system: dizziness, sleepiness, vertigo

Other: back pain, headache

OVERDOSAGE

There is no experience in humans with overdosage. Acute oral toxicity studies in animals, however, using doses up to 12 gm/kg body weight, could not find a lethal dose. Risks associated with overdosage should, therefore, be minimal.

DOSAGE AND ADMINISTRATION

Active Duodenal Ulcer: The recommended adult oral dosage for duodenal ulcer is 1 gm four times a day on an empty stomach.

Antacids may be prescribed as needed for relief of pain but should not be taken within one-half hour before or after sucralfate.

While healing with sucralfate may occur during the first week or two, treatment should be continued for 4 to 8 weeks unless healing has been demonstrated by x-ray or endoscopic examination.

Maintenance Therapy: The recommended adult oral dosage is 1 gm twice a day.

HOW SUPPLIED

CARAFATE (sucralfate) 1-gm tablets are supplied in bottles of 100 (NDC 0088-1712-47), 120 (NDC 0088-1712-53), and 500 (NDC 0088-1712-55) and in Unit Dose Identification Paks of 100 (NDC 0088-1712-49). Light pink scored oblong tablets are embossed with CARAFATE on one side and 1712 bracketed by C's on the other.

Issued 4/90

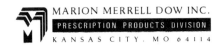
MARION MERRELL DOW INC.
PRESCRIPTION PRODUCTS DIVISION
KANSAS CITY, MO 64114